To my cousin
Wesley W. Rees
with deepest
gratitude and love,
Naomi Turner
Aug. 16, 1980

# I REMEMBER—

To

Linda, Deborah, Peter, Frederick,
Janine, Elizabeth and Caroline

# I REMEMBER—

by

PROFESSOR C. E. TURNER

*Professor of Public Health Emeritus, Masachusetts Institute of Technology; Honorary President, International Union for Health Education; Recipient of the Medaille d'Or, of the National Academy of Medicine of France and of the Grosse Verdienstkreuz of the West German Republic; Formerly Chief of Health Education, World Health Organization; Sometime Associate Professor of Hygiene, Tufts Medical and Dental Schools; and Visiting Professor of Health Education, School of Public Health, University of California.*

VANTAGE PRESS

NEW YORK WASHINGTON HOLLYWOOD

FIRST EDITION



Published by Vantage Press, Inc
516 West 34th Street, New York, N. Y. 10001

Manufactured in the United States of America

Standard Book No. 533-00931-6

## PREFACE

This book is not the story of my life. It is a recounting of a variety of experiences.

My arrival in a village of about 25 houses and 100 people was on the morning of April 28, 1890, at the age of zero hours. My mother was 29 years old and my father 35. He was the village doctor.

Some of the memories reported here reflect the sharp contrasts between life in the 1890's and in the 1970's. Other memories tell about things that happened for the first time in health or in education. Still others describe interesting people or unusual experiences.

C. E. T.
Arlington, Mass.
April 1973

## CONTENTS

# 1

## VILLAGE LIFE IN THE 1890'S

Many pioneer families in colonial days lived four or five miles from the nearest neighbor. Life for a boy in a Maine village of 100 people in the 1890's was not quite like that, but it was nearer like pioneer living than it was like life in today's cities. People lived in single-family houses with no apartment buildings anywhere. In most families there were grandparents, and often there were aunts and uncles. We knew everyone in the village, and most days we saw no one whom we did not know. The house and barn were never locked at night.

One of the greatest gifts to boys and girls of the twentieth century has been music. Music is always available to you. Great music, sweet music, jazz, rock—music from many times and from many places. You can hardly imagine days before radio, television, records and cassettes. We had only such music as members of the family or community could make. Any country boy or girl who really loved music was music-starved in those days.

Apparently in the 1880's most Maine towns had had a brass band, but in my memory the village bandstand was the only relic of ours. My mother was a member of a women's quartet which sang in church and at entertainments. In the parlor we had an organ which was pumped with foot pedals. There were more organs than pianos in town. I was given lessons on the organ, and I remember the teacher and her pointer with which she used to rap my fingers.

The lack of real music promoted the use of harmonicas, jews' harps and noise-makers such as wooden rib-shaped "bones" and homemade whistles. The growing layer of certain plants like the alder bush is very soft in the spring. By hammering lightly a branch the size of one's finger, a section of bark could be slipped off. The wood beneath it was then cut like the parts of a whistle. The bark was slipped back and a notch made at the proper place.

In those days before the movies, entertainments were limited and mostly "homemade." Each year in our village a local play was produced under the leadership of my mother and two or three other energetic people. There would be a period of several weeks of rehearsals, then presentation of the play in our village, followed by a hayride trip for the group to one or two other villages to present the play.

About once a year there would be what was called a Kickapoo Indian Medicine Show. Why they used the name "Kickapoo" I do not know, because the Kickapoos were originally of Wisconsin, then moved to Oklahoma. I suppose it was the charm of the word which caused it to be so used. The show stayed two or three days in the village. At their evening shows they sold bottles of "medicine." I do not know what it was, but I suspect it was water in which some roots had been boiled. They also sold small cakes of soap which produced fabulous quantities of lather.

The standard social activities were the truly remarkable suppers given by the local Grange or by either the Methodist or Baptist Church. What a saliva-stimulating sight those long white tables presented to hungry boys! Whipped-cream layer cakes with pieces of red jelly on the top; other cakes with white sugar frosting covered with tiny candies; apple pies; pumpkin pies; pitchers of milk!

And then there was the Christmas tree in the church which was attended by just about everyone. The huge tree was trimmed mainly with popcorn strung on threads, with pine cones, and with such other decorations as the community afforded. A Santa Claus in a fur coat came in with a pack of presents and read the names of the happy recipients.

This activity meant a great deal to all of us. I know because my parents later told me that, when I was at the age of about seven, they thought I was too much concerned with what I would get at Christmas and told me, "This year you may not get so much." They apparently did a good job in the telling, because I almost completely lost my appetite and decided I would not go to the Christmas tree. The therapy was as clearcut as the etiology. My mother said, "Go along to the Christmas tree. You'll probably get as much as anybody"—after which there was no trace of the malady.

What could a boy do in those days? Actually, life was far from dull. Any boy with three horses, a dog, a bicycle, a fishpole, a sled, and a pair of snowshoes did not lack for something to do. Trout-fishing was good in the early summer. Many of the farmers in our town tapped maple trees in the spring and boiled down the maple syrup. In springtime the sun melted the snowdrifts at the top, and the freezing temperature at night formed a crust on the snowdrifts so hard that one could run or slide upon it. Two or three of us boys together would hike a mile or two outside the village to the maple grove and syrup house of some farmer. Hot cream-of-tartar biscuits with newly-made maple syrup was one of the best possible ways to quench hiking-induced hunger.

One of the greatest contrasts between the 1890's and the 1970's has been in the practice of medicine. My father kept three horses pretty tired in driving many miles every day, seven days a week; but my first personal experience with medical care came when I broke my arm.

At the age of seven or eight I received my bicycle. Apparently kid-size bikes were not available. Anyhow, mine did not allow my feet to reach the pedals; so the village blacksmith put on pedal extensions. I was learning to ride on a Sunday morning when the bicycle went out from under me and my left arm was broken at the elbow. My father was, of course, the only doctor within twenty miles, and he was some eight or ten miles away making house calls. There were no telephones and the only way to reach him was to send someone after him. Fortunately he had left word as to where he was going, and the neighbor across the street hitched up another one of our horses and started after my father. He thought he knew where to go; he checked his travels by asking at an occasional farmhouse, "Have you seen the doctor go by today?"

It was about three hours after I broke my arm when my father got home. I remember taking ether, but I do not know if anyone helped father in administering it, in setting the arm, and in applying the plaster-of-paris cast.

In such an accident today a child would be taken to the emergency room of a hospital. X-rays would show the doctors the exact condition of the broken bone, and a doctor would not have to treat his own child. Father had no X-ray, and he was certainly anxious about this break in the elbow lest it leave me with a stiff arm.

As in my case, any person with severe illness or accident in a country village had only a general practitioner of medicine as a medical resource. Neither trained nurses nor practical nurses were available, although a few women in the community had gained some skill in caring for the sick and could be called upon in very serious emergencies. The nearest dentist was twenty-two miles away. The physician had to order drugs from a drug house in the city. Father carried in the buggy or sleigh a medicine case with solid walls containing vials of pills, powder, or liquid. He also had a soft leather bag which carried surgical instruments.

Today a patient may receive the attention of any one of more than a dozen medical specialists. The physician or surgeon has the assistance of registered nurses, practical nurses, nurses' aides, anesthetists, physical therapists, dieticians, pharmacists, radiologists, laboratory and other technicians. Your imagination pictures the problems of the sick in getting medical care a century ago. It can also paint pictures for you of the labors, efforts and frustrations of the country doctor confronted with a limitless variety of medical ailments and restricted medical resources.

# 2

## WHEN A DOLLAR WAS A DOLLAR

Money was hard to come by in rural Maine in the 1890's. We were not poor; we just didn't have any money.

I recall that in father's medical-practice office calls were fifty cents. The rewards for labor (skilled in varying degrees) were very low. We usually had a "hired girl" who was paid $2.50 a week and a "hired man" or "chore boy" who was given $30.00 a month and board. The term "maid" and "hostler" were not used, as they were much too fancy, "high-falutin'," and undemocratic to be socially acceptable. There was no loss of status in "hiring out" on such jobs. The hired man and hired girl ate with the family. They were from farm families, and usually married eventually and lived on a farm or went away to work in the city.

Our town was entirely given over to farming. There were no other jobs except one at the general store, one at the little hotel, one at the grain mill, and one at a small mill for spinning yarn which was operated by a man and his son. In 1901 the railroad came to our village and a creamery was built. There, butterfat was separated from the milk brought in from the farms, and shipped as cream to the city.

My own first job was when I "hired out in haying" at the age of fourteen for a dollar a day and board. I remember how heavy the hand scythe seemed and the effort needed to keep ahead of the farmer (age fifty, weight 200 pounds) who was mowing the swath behind me. Our chief staple food was boiled potatoes with slices of fat pork swimming in its own "tried-out" fat in a bowl. We had lean meat only once in the two weeks and that was by "accident." At least, I have always maintained that it was an accident.

You see, it happened this way. The farmer had a flock of about twenty hens. In the daytime they often gathered in the yard in front of the barn door. On this particular day they were there when I came up from the field to hitch the old gray mare to the horse rake. She was ordinarily steady enough, but for some (unexplained) reason she wheeled suddenly to the left and the right wheel rolled through a clump of a half-dozen hens and over the neck of one of them. My hunger for meat outweighed my compassion for an animal. I grabbed up the hen, climbed back onto the seat of the horse rake, and threw old Dolly into high gear toward the field where the farmer was working. "Damn fool hen had to get run over!" said he. "Only thing to do is to kill her, dress her, and have her for dinner tomorrow."

But if wages were low, so was the cost of living. Milk was 5 cents a quart; potatoes, 30 cents a bushel. Bread was baked at home, but when it first appeared in our stores at the turn of the century it was 5 cents a loaf. (I saw a special advertisement yesterday outside our supermarket for first-quality bread at 89 cents a loaf; and bread will be still more expensive before this story reaches you.)

The man who lived next door to us was an old soldier living on a Civil War pension of thirty dollars a month. He and his wife and one son managed very well on that plus what came from having a garden, a cow and a few hens. I recall that he did not smoke or drink or keep a horse and carriage.

The first concentration of wealth which came to my attention involved a largely retired older man who sat in the general store much of the time and from whom, in the absence of a bank of any kind, our good citizens could borrow money at 6% secured by a mortgage covering a new house or an expected crop. He had no farm although he may have had one once. He did buy wool from the farmers every spring and ship it to market. His first name was Richard, and he was always known as "Rich Marble." I don't know how rich he really was, but in those days a man who had $20,000 and owned his own home was regarded as being really "well off." He could live quite comfortably on the interest of $1,200 a year. There were no income taxes and there were no inheritance taxes, so whatever he "died possessed of" went to his children.

Real-estate taxes were very low. Our taxes on a house, woodshed, carriage house and stable with three or four horses was around $25 or $35 a year; and these were our only taxes. As late as 1911 the tax on the clubhouse and three other buildings, plus 1500 acres of lakeshore and woodland owned by a sportsman's club of out-of-state members in our town, was only $150.

But even then taxes had been going up ever since the incorporation of the town in 1803. A paragraph regarding the payment of taxes from the record of the town meeting in 1811 reads as follows: "Voted $200 for the support of schools and received in pay corn at 5 shillings, rye at six shillings and wheat at seven shillings per bushel. Voted $800 on the highway to be paid in labor of men and oxen at 12½¢ an hour."

There was no national debt. As I write this in 1968 the press is saying that "the interest on the national debt for the coming year will be more than 16 billion." (*U.S. News,* May 13, 1968, p. 26.) This is over $80 for every man, woman and child, or $400 for a family of five.

# 3

## HEATING AND LIGHTING

I remember the cold dark winters in Maine in the 1890's.

Breakfast was at seven. That meant that we got up in the dark. First I would strike a match and light a kerosene oil lamp, then hurry into some "fleece-lined" underwear, thick woolen stockings, woolen trousers, and buckle rubber boots in place of shoes.

How cold it was! As soon as the lamp was lighted I could see my breath when breathing out. There was only one warm room in the house in the morning in those days of wood stoves. Let me explain.

In the time of deep snow every winter the farmers who sold wood would cut down some birch and maple trees, then chop the trunk and large limbs into sled-lengths of about ten feet. We bought a few cords. It was loaded onto horse sleds, hauled to our back yard and piled up alongside the wood shed.

Sometimes it was sawed up by a man with a bucksaw or the big sticks were sawed by two men using a crosscut saw. A much more exciting procedure was sawing it by machine. This was a two-horsepower machine, common in those days before the internal combustion engine. Steam engines were of course in use on the railroad, but there were no portable engines in country towns. Power was generated by a horse-operated treadmill. The horses were big and friendly, weighing some 1500 to 1600 pounds each. They were led into the treadmill and the brake was released. The sloping plank floor of the treadmill began to roll backward and the horses began walking. The big wheel attached to the treadmill began to turn. A long leather belt from the wheel ran to another and much smaller wheel on the shaft which carried the circular saw. As the saw picked up speed it was ready to cut the wood into stove lengths as the long sticks were laid on the cradle and pressed against it.

After the wood was in stove lengths it had to be split for the cook-stove, and some was left unsplit for the big stove in the living room. The hired man spent part of each fair day of February and March splitting wood.

Of course the fire in the kitchen stove went out every night because the fire box would not hold enough wood to burn more than three or four hours. But the big iron stove in the living room was something else again. It was about the size of a small barrel and had a heavy iron base. It would take a stick of hard wood which was as big as the biggest grocery bag and as heavy as a ten-year-old boy could carry. (We used to say it was all he could lug.) After the stick was burning well the stove was closed up and the fire burned slowly through the night.

But I started to tell you about light in those days. We still had a few candles in case the village store ran out of kerosene, and we also had a candle mold to make our own. The mold was a frame with six hollow cylinders, each the shape of a candle. A cotton wick was hung along the center of each cylinder and melted mutton tallow was poured in around it and allowed to harden.

But except in emergency we used kerosene lamps. (Thomas Edison had invented the incandescent light in 1879; but electric power and electric lights were still some years away in our village.)

Kerosene was about 10 cents to 14 cents a gallon. When we heard of a gift of John D. Rockefeller to one of his favorite charities, it was standard local humor to say that the price of kerosene would go up a cent a gallon.

The kind of lamp I remember best was the "hand lamp." Each person carried one with him in going from room to room. In the morning the lamps were brought to the kitchen and set in a row along the shelf beside the kitchen sink. The size of their yellow flame could be increased by turning up the wick, and the chimney of each lamp was almost sure to accumulate some smoke from the burning oil. After the breakfast dishes were washed the hired girl spent an hour trimming wicks, washing the chimneys, and filling the lamps with oil.

There was also a lantern to be cleaned and filled. Lamps were so difficult to carry and to set down that the lantern with its wire bale handle and broad base was used in doing evening and before-breakfast chores in the barn. In the winter the horses were fed after dark and before daylight.

BAIL

At the other cultural extreme was the parlor lamp. This was indeed a thing of magnificence. The lamp proper was a metal oil container topped by a wick holder which supported a glass chimney. But none of these were visible to the admiring onlooker. The metal lamp was enclosed in a porcelain globe and another such globe covered the glass chimney. These globes were hand-painted, and the mellow light shining through the upper globe bathed the parlor in a glow of mixed opulence and hospitality.

By modern standards our house was dark and (unless one sat rather close to a stove) a bit cold in mid-winter. But to us it was cheerful, light, and cozy-warm. In those pre-electricity days of the 1890's the wood-burning stoves and the kerosene lamps were the only service appliances in addition to chairs, tables, beds, and other furniture in the homes of those of us who lived in rural Maine. No wonder that we valued them highly!

# 4

## THE KITCHEN WAS THE HEADQUARTERS OF THE HOUSEHOLD

There were two times in the week when a small boy was sure to be in the kitchen. One was when doughtnuts were being fried and one was when loaves of raised bread were coming out of the oven of the big wood-burning cook-stove.

Altogether our kitchen was a remarkable room. It had six doors. On the north side, one door opened into the front hall and another into the cellarway. On the south side one doorway led to the pantry in which food was prepared and another one into the shed. The door on the east opened into the master bedroom and the door on the west into the dining room.

There were two other rooms on the first floor. The one at the front or north side of the house was the "office" where father saw clinical patients. This opened into the front hall and the master bedroom. The other room was the parlor which opened into the front hall and into the dining room.

At one side of the cook-stove was a woodbox which I had to keep filled by bringing in wood from the shed. My grandmother said I should never come in without bringing an armful of wood. We had a "generation gap" on that subject.

On the other side of the stove was an iron sink with a small hand pump which brought water from a well outside the house. Over the sink was a long shelf which held the half-dozen small kerosene hand lamps.

In those days very few prepared foods were available; and the prevention of food spoilage was a rather elaborate process, differing quite sharply in summer and in winter. We did not need any refrigeration in the winter to provide freezing temperatures because those temperatures existed consistently in the washroom and sheds outside the kitchen door. Each November we either had a fattened hog to kill or bought a whole hog which was dressed, cut up, and packed in a big chest in the shed. Usually father brought home a deer in the fall hunting season. Much of the deer meat was used in making mincemeat for pies, and the steaks were put in the freezer chest.

Nothing like the present prime western beef was available. There was a butcher's wagon or sled which came around once a week. The beef was native grown and not well fattened. The sheep, lamb or pork which the butcher brought was of medium quality.

In the summertime the whole picture was changed. Food was kept cool in an ice chest. The top of this chest lifted up to receive a cake of ice about 18 by 12 by 12 inches in size. The food was put in a little cupboard below the ice box and the two compartments were connected by air passages. Ice had to be put in the ice chest every day or every other day, depending on the weather. The ice chest drained into a pan which had to be emptied daily.

There was no iceman in our village, which meant that we had to harvest our own ice. We had a separate ice house which was filled each winter. This little house had floor space about 12 by 15 feet. When the ice on the millpond at the foot of the hill had frozen to a depth of 15 to 24 inches, the ice harvesting took place. The cakes were marked by a horsedrawn cutter and cut by a man with a crosscut saw with a handle only at one end. The cakes which he cut were some 18 or 20 inches square. They were pulled out of the water, loaded on a sled, and hauled up to the ice house, into which they were packed in a mound of ice some six feet high. This mound was covered with sawdust which filled in the space between the ice and the walls. The sawdust over the top of the ice was nearly a foot thick. It was quite a process to get a piece of ice from the ice house, get the sawdust cleanly washed off, then get the ice placed in the ice chest.

Many families in the village did not harvest ice, but kept food as best they could on the cool floor of the cellar. These were the days of increasing demand for refrigeration. Cutting ice on the Kennebec River and shipping it to Boston and New York by railroad freight cars was an important business in Maine. It seems strange now to think of the days when the water in big rivers was sufficiently clean and unpolluted to make the harvesting and family use of ice possible.

The arrival of electric refrigerators and the making of artificial ice put an end to the ice-harvesting industry, just as the development of concrete and macadam for road-making put an end to the cutting of stone paving blocks along the Maine Coast. That was also a big business in the 1890's. Granite cliffs at the water's edge were developed into quarries from which paving blocks were cut and loaded onto scows which could be brought into the shallow water at the shore. The scows were then pulled out to deep water and the stones transferred to three-masted sailing vessels for shipment to cities. Even today one finds an occasional bit of street paved with stone in some cities.

Another food repository of great importance was the doughnut jar, an earthen crock which was always kept on the second stair of the cellarway. I was allowed to lunch on doughnuts, but I remember that the hired girl was constantly unhappy because doughnuts disappeared from the doughnut crock so quickly. There were also shelves for food over the cellar stairs. Vegetables were not bought from week to week, but one or two bushels of potatoes, beets, carrots and turnips were bought in the fall and stored in the vegetable closet of the cellar.

The kitchen was in a sense also the headquarters for the cleanliness operations of the household. In these pre-electricity days dishes were washed by hand in the sink after each meal. Clothes were washed in the washroom or shed just outside the kitchen in the summertime, but in cold winter weather the washtubs were brought into the kitchen. I remember bars of yellow laundry soap and also a hogshead of semi-liquid soft soap at the bottom of the cellar stairs. The soft soap was made from lye and pork fat. The lye was made by draining water through a pail of wood ashes. The fats were accumulated from food scraps and digested in the lye to form soap.

Such were some of the laborious activities of the kitchen and the household in the days before electric heating, electric lighting, electric washing, and electric refrigeration.

# 5

## THE YEARS OF THE HORSE

Have you ever thought of the limited movement of people before the days of the automobile, paved streets and blacktop roads? Your car is ready to go whenever you step into it. If you wish, you drive a mile a minute for 100 to 600 miles in a day. In the time of the dirt road in northern New England, there was an extra season called "mud-time." The horse carried one at eight or ten miles an hour, preferably for not more than twenty miles a day.

Not every family had a horse. Most farmers had work horses, although oxen were still used for much of the heavy work. On the farm it did not cost much to keep a horse, so a driving horse was usually kept in addition. In our village there were perhaps fifteen or twenty horses. Of the nine families on our street only two had horses. Father, as a doctor, usually kept three. The family across the street had a pair of workhorses because they farmed several acres.

The care of the horses was a major function of the hired man. Three times a day he backed them out of their stalls and led them to the watering trough for a drink. In the morning before we had our breakfast, he went up to the hayloft above the horses' stalls and pushed some hay through the hole in the hayloft floor in front of each horse. He also brought oats from the granary for the horses' breakfast. Similarly, he provided a noon meal and a supper for the animals. He kept the stalls clean and he also fed the cow and the hogs regularly.

Each horse had to be curried and brushed daily. It had its own harness which was kept soft and fit by occasional washing with harness soap and rubbing with oil. In the winter the harnesses were frozen stiff, and the steel bit for the horse's mouth had to be warmed in one's hands before the bridle was put on to avoid the horse's tongue getting stuck to the cold metal.

I remember particularly a bad winter storm in which the wind howled and blew the snow into drifts all night. The next morning drifts were more than waist-high across the road in front of our house. It was beautiful to look at, but distressing to a physician who had seriously-ill patients miles away. About eleven o'clock in the morning the farmers from the North Road got into the village with the "breaking-out team," consisting of four yoke of oxen pulling a sled with a birch log under the front runners. That sort of treatment opened up the roads somewhat, but they were still almost impassable.

In the afternoon, father had to see some patients. Two road-horses, Dick and Plum, were hooked up tandem to a wide-runnered sled. Dick was the front horse and he would plow through the drifts. Plum, also in harness and close behind him, would draw the sled. The medicine case and satchel of surgical instruments which represented the doctor's limited resources were put in the front of the sled. The back of the sled had rather a large open space which carried a pair of snowshoes, because there was always the chance that even the tandem team could not make it and that the horses must be left at a farm barn while the doctor snowshoed the last few miles.

Our mail ordinarily came once a day by horse-drawn stage from the railhead twelve miles away. At the time of this storm the roads were completely blocked for several days. On the third day after the storm a man brought the mail sack on snowshoes.

You wonder where were the now-ubiquitous skiis? The first ones I saw were after the turn of the century when a Norwegian family moved into town. Snowshoes were plentiful. They had been made by the Indians before and during the earliest days of the colonies.

Every child that grew up in the country in the days of the horse had his adventures with them. I remember at the age of about eight taking a buggy some twelve or fifteen miles to get it painted. Going down I had a gig attached to the back of the wagon, and coming back I rode in the gig. In today's methods of transportation an eight-year-old has little chance of such an adventure by himself.

The rural East of the country was quite different from the West in horseback riding. It did exist, but was somewhat unusual. At about a dozen years of age, I received a McClellan saddle; and I well remember my first adventure in it. The hired man cinched up the saddle. I mounted and started up the road to find out suddenly that a horse which had never been ridden and a boy who had never been on a horse before produced a somewhat unpropitious combination. Dick, my horse, started to run, and everything was going well until suddenly I saw ahead of us a tank truck of kerosene hauled by two pair of heavy horses and taking up most of the width of the narrow country road. My horse jumped the ditch at the right, jumped a very low stone wall into the field, ran on by the truck, and then jumped back into the road, with me clinging most unmanfully to the front of the saddle.

Some of the time, but not always, we had a cow; and always we had hogs in a space under the barn and extending into an outside pen. I remember particularly a period of a few years when I was six or eight years old when we had a boar of good ancestry. He was a strong, sturdy fellow with long tusks and a formidable expression. He was very strong, and on two or three occasions he got his nose under the fence in the outside yard, lifted the fence, and ran out.

Having grown up away from hogs, you are unaware of the difficulty for one small boy to drive a hog into a barn. With some fear, I adopted a technique which relied upon hunger. I filled a pint measure with whole corn of a coarse, red variety. Getting fairly near to the boar, I threw a handful of corn on the ground. He came forward and ate it, and

I began backing up toward the open barn doors, scattering corn along the way. He followed me into the barn, eating the corn. I put a handful in the middle of the floor, and while he was eating it I closed the barn doors.

But then the problem was how to get him back into the pen. There was a trapdoor in the cow's stall. This I lifted out and put a handful of corn at the edge of the hole. While the boar was facing the hole in the floor and eating the corn, I rushed the unsuspecting gentleman from the rear and gave him a sudden unexpected push into the hole in the floor and down into the pen. To a small boy this was an adventure in danger and an achievement.

At the age of about eight I was assigned some of the chores to do, and year by year such assigned duties were increased. I am sorry that there were no such duties for you living in town in the nuclear family, because such assignments had an urgency about them. Where there were animals to be cared for, there was not only insistence on the part of parents that the chores be done promptly and well; there was also the knowledge that animals, of which one was very fond, would suffer if they were not fed, watered, and cared for regularly.

# 6

# BUFFALO BILL

Some time between the ages of six and nine—I am not sure just when—my father took me to Bangor to see Buffalo Bill's Wild West Show. During the years 1895 to 1899, Colonel Cody's show was becoming famous. I do not know whether he came to Maine more than once.

It was early in the morning when my father came to the foot of the stairs and shouted, "Son, Buffalo Bill's show is in Bangor. Would you like to go see it?" You can imagine the speed with which I dressed and came downstairs. We drove to the rail terminus and did the 50-mile train trip to Bangor. I cannot remember much about the trip or staying in the hotel overnight, but I do remember the thrill of the father-and-son trip and I have most vivid recollections of the show itself.

The tent was rectangular in shape. Or I should say that the tent flanked three sides of a rectangular space. The horsemen came in from the rear. Our seats were in the front row at the front end of the seating space. Different groups of horsemen came in and rode twice around the enclosure. They were cavalry units, Indians, and cowboys. Each group stopped in front of the seats where we were sitting, and as a new group came in, the groups already there backed their horses away from us.

Finally, when all the mounted riders were in place, Buffalo Bill rode in amidst great applause, stopped his horse in front of the other horsemen, and lifted his white sombrero as his horse reared spectacularly. I remember also the trick riding and the "attack" on a stagecoach by a band of supposed Indians as the stagecoach was driven around and around the enclosure. It was eventually "liberated" by a supposed cavalry unit. There was also the shooting of glass balls thrown into the air.

Colonel Cody lived until 1917, but his summer tours of small cities were primarily in the 90's. Whatever his contributions may have been in interpreting the early days of the West rightly and wrongly, the show undoubtedly cemented many father-son relationships.

I had another indirect contact with Buffalo Bill's Wild West. When I was teaching in Hawaii during the summer of 1930, one of the school people who knew of my interest in Hawaiian history arranged for me to meet a Mrs. Mokamier, a retired schoolteacher. She was a lady then about eighty years of age. As a young man, her husband had been for two or three years with Buffalo Bill. Having a dark skin, he passed as an Indian, but was really a full-blooded Hawaiian.

After his trouping with Buffalo Bill, Mr. Mokamier, still a young man, returned to Honolulu and became a member of the police force. Mrs. Mokamier told me of one of his surprising experiences. The missionaries felt that the Hawaiians should be married in the Christian faith, and so the police were asked to go up the valley and bring down all of the old people who had families of grown children in order that they might enjoy a Christian wedding. Mrs. Mokamier told me that her husband did not mind asking his father to come down, but he was terribly embarrassed to ask his mother. However, both parents took it as a joke and rode down to town in a big wagon with their neighbors.

Mrs. Mokamier told me also of the ancient custom by which each year runners for the king went over the island and selected eight or ten of the most beautiful teenage girls to live in the palace for a year to grace the court before returning to their respective villages. This was a great honor; and they and their children were the only persons who could stand in the presence of the king, as the custom was for the people to drop to their knees when the king appeared. Mr. Mokamier's mother had been so honored.

# 7

## LOCAL MAINE HUMOR

In the days before populations became so mobile, country towns cherished and passed on from generation to generation humorous remarks or situations with which their citizens had been involved. In many cases these stories had a bit of philosophy as well as a bit of humor.

There was, for example, the story of Philander Parkman's unplanted field. A fellow townsman driving by in mid-July saw Philander sitting on his front porch and stopped to ask, "What are you going to do with that acre of plowed land I just drove by?"

"Gracious," said Philander, "I forgot all about it. I was going to plant it to potatoes." After a brief contemplative pause he continued, "Oh, well! You can't think of everything in one spring."

It was always reassuring to remember Philander's philosophy when one forgot something.

Then there is the story of the man who was hauling food supplies to a lumber camp in Northern Penobscot County when he met a lone lumberjack walking south.

"Where are you going?" inquired the teamster.

The lumberjack replied, "I'm going to Bangor to get drunk, and Gad, how I dread it!"

Another story is that of the college professor who was spending his summer in a village in Somerset County and who needed to go to the county seat to look up a deed. He engaged the livery man to drive him to the shire town. As they were going down a hill, the strap that attached the breeching to the back strap gave way. (As you may know, the breeching is a broad strap that goes before the wagon and behind the horse and keeps the wagon from running onto the animal going downhill.) The livery man stopped at the next farm and got the owner to tie up the harness with a small piece of rope. As he finished the professor enquired, "Will this emergency apparatus meet the exigencies of the situation?"

"Huh?" said the farmer.

"He means," said the livery man, "will the damn thing hold till we get to Skowhegan."

We liked stories of keen repartee, like the story of the witty lawyer of small physical stature who was badgered by the opposing lawyer of 6'2" and 212 lbs. At the end of this lawyer's oration he said to his diminutive opponent, "Squire, I could put you in my pocket."

"If you did," was the reply, "You'd have more law in your pocket than you have in your head."

Seems like everybody in southern Somerset County knew the story of Rill Smart and the Squire.

Rill was a working man. (Less considerate people of today would have called him a laborer.) The Squire was a well-to-do retired lawyer and the local judge. They met early one summer morning on the main road running through the village.

"Good morning, Rillius," said the Squire.

"Good morning, Squire," said Rill. "Why are you out so early?"

"Why Rillius," was the reply, "I'm after an appetite for my breakfast. Why are you out so early?"

"Hell," said Rill, "I am after a breakfast for my appetite!"

We liked to repeat that actual bit of drama, perhaps because it seemed to smack of Yankee democracy with economic differences.

There was the story of Mr. Quimby and the eggs which illustrated man's anxiety to avoid losing face.

In those days the village storekeeper engaged in barter. Eggs were a crop which could be exchanged for groceries;

and such a transaction is just what Mr. Q. had in mind that morning when he set a pail of eggs on the grocery counter.

"Are these strictly fresh?" asked the grocer.

"Absolutely, every one of them has been laid since noon yesterday," said Mr. Quimby, with a lift of the chin and a squaring of the shoulders which should make clear his resentment that such a question could even be asked of a man of his business integrity.

The storekeeper took the eggs into the back room where eggs were stored and, because he had a good balance of perspicacity and credulity, he candled them to determine their quality. He came back to the customer with two eggs in the pail.

"I'm sorry, Mr. Quimby," he said, "two of these eggs are not good."

What an awkward situation for Mr. Quimby! The two eggs were certainly bad—he was free to check them for himself. He stared at the two eggs in the pail as several thoughts raced through his mind. Why this surprise tactic of checking the quality of eggs? City folks should expect to get a bad egg now and then. Bringing in eggs of varying freshness was not such a sin. But then his thought returned to his own exact words certifying their freshness. After a long and somewhat awkward pause he closed the incident with the words, "Well, all I can say is: Damn a hen that will lay a rotten egg."

Like any reasonably homogeneous racial and cultural group, we in our town were comfortably satisfied with ourselves and we were somewhat disturbed by outsiders, even though they did not come from very far out. Every summer we boys were expected to add a few city kids to our vacation activities. They loved to tell us about trolley cars, theatres, and other things we had never seen. When we were fed up with one of these kids, we lost him in the woods for an hour or so.

A fair number of adult vacationers came to our area. Our chatty stage driver was taking one of them back to the train when cultural differences got into the conversation.

"I'll say one thing for Maine. You have a lot of 'queer' people around here," said the returning urbanite.

"Yes," said the stage driver, "they are coming and going on every train this time of year."

There is another story of this kind which originated down on the coast, but for the accuracy of which I cannot vouch.

As the story goes, a squall came up suddenly one day and tipped over a sailboat manned by one of the "natives," who died of heart failure. Next day two lobster fishermen were discussing the accident. "Bill, your boat was on the other side of the harbor," said Tom. "Why didn't you go across to help him?"

"I feel awful bad about that," said Bill. "But at the time I thought he was a summer visitor."

Almost as characteristic of the psychological group defense mechanism against outsiders reflected in the stories just recorded were the poems we children were required to memorize for the frequent occasions when we had to "speak pieces." People probably felt their isolation and the need to make clear our important place in society.

I recall the story told by a poem which described a family of three farm boys. The two older boys went away to school, but the one who stayed home got to be Governor.

There were two poems I memorized to recite at the last day of school exercises over seventy years ago. One poem told of a wonderful Fourth of July celebration in a rural town. It began:

> Old Ripton was a Yankee town amid the fair green
>   mountains,
> Where woodland streams came leaping down, from
>   sparkling springs and fountains.
> Where seldom with the world outside
>   Her rustic genius mingled,
> Where men were mostly occupied
>   In making staves and shingles.

The glorious Fourth of each July
  Was made a grand occasion,
Each patriot put his business by,
  To swell the celebration.

The poem that I remember best, and which was the most provincial, was "The Yankee in the Catacombs." I was compelled to memorize it during the golden age of ten or eleven when things committed to memory stay with one for life, almost in their completeness. As I remember it, and have repeated it to my grandchildren, it says:

Never lived a Yankee yet but was ready to bet on
  the U.S.A.
If you spoke of Italy's sunny clime, Maine could
  beat it every time.
If you spoke of Aetna's Mound of Fire, you would
  raise his ire,
And in an injured way he would probably say,
"I don't think much of a smokin' hill, but we got a
  moderate little rill
That would make your old volcano still.
Just pour old Niagara down the crater, guess that
  would soothe her fiery natur'."
Sam Jones was a fellow from way down East who never
  was staggered in the least.
No wondrous tale of beast or bird could match
  the stories he had heard.
No wondrous sight or curious view was equal to
  Podunk, I tell you.
They showed him a room where a queen had slept—
  " 'Twan't up to the tavern Daddy kept."
They showed him Lucerne; but he had drunk from the
  beautiful Molly Chunckamunk.
At last they took him to ancient Rome and inveigled
  him into a catacomb.
Here they plied him with draughts of wine, though

he vowed old cider was twice as fine,
Till the fumes of Falernia filled his head, and he
slept as still as the silent dead.
They moved a mummy to give him room and laid him
at length in the rocky tomb.
They piled old skeletons round the stone, set a dip
in a candlestick of bone,
And left him to slumber there alone,
Watching from a distance the tapers gleam, ready
to jeer at his frightened scream
When he should awake from his drunken dream.
After a time the Yankee awoke, but instantly saw
through the flimsy joke.
So never a shout or a cry he uttered, but solemnly rose
and slowly muttered,
"I see how 'tis, it's the Judgment Day. We have all
been dead and stowed away;
All you foreigners sleeping yet? I'm the first one
up, you bet.
Can't none of you fellows start, I wonder,
United States ahead, by thunder."

# 8

## SCHOOLS AND SCHOOLING

In the 19th century the town of Harmony had no high school and no grade school. The village school and the district schools outside the village had a fall term and a spring term of nine or ten weeks each, taught usually by a young woman whose preparation beyond seven years in these very schools consisted of two years in one of the state normal schools.

One of my earliest educational remembrances is that of being "read to" by the hour by a friend of my mother. Aunt May Dore was the widow of a Union soldier. She lived in a second-floor apartment in a building occupied by the owner, who mended harnesses. His wife was a dressmaker. I remember lying on Aunt May's rug on the floor, and I was told later that my constant request at the slightest pause was, "Read, Aunt May, read."

The books were mostly those of the English war correspondent and writer G. A. Henty, who seems to have written a book at the small-boy level concerning most of the major wars recorded in history, under such titles as "With Lee in Virginia," "With Clive in India," and "With Frederick the Great."

My first half-day of school placed me in basic opposition to the establishment and the whole educational process. It happened that the teacher that fall was a young man. I do not know his preparation for teaching. I do remember that he was the pitcher on the village baseball team. I was enjoying my front seat by tipping my head straight back to see how far behind me I could see the ceiling. Suddenly a textbook landed on my desk and slid against my abdomen, bringing me upright with a start—a credit to the pitching ability of the teacher. At noon I told my parents that schools might be all right for some kids but I had had enough. Father said, "You march yourself back there, young man"; and I have been in the education business ever since.

My ungraded village school usually had fifteen to twenty pupils from six to thirteen years of age and confined itself mainly to the 3 R's, with some geography plus a little grammar and English composition. We had Scripture-reading and prayer every morning at the opening of school. The pupils were all Wasps (white, Anglo-Saxon and Protestant), bearing such names as Perkins, Newmarch, Bartlet, Bailey, Hatch, Herrick, Rhoades and Turner.

We had no music, except that sometimes we sang without accompaniment. We had no physical education. At recess we played "haley-over" by throwing a rubber ball over the schoolhouse. We chose sides, and the side which threw the ball shouted "Haley over!" when they threw it. Someone on the other team caught the ball and everyone ran around the end of the schoolhouse, the boy or girl with the ball trying not to get caught.

Or we played Coram. A space in the schoolyard about fifty or sixty feet wide was marked off by poles laid on the ground. One boy or girl who was a good runner stood back of one pole and all the other children stood back of the other one. The lone boy shouted, "Coram!" All the others started across the measured strip, and he caught whomsoever he could. The caught pupils joined the catching team and this process continued until all were caught.

Or we dammed up a pool in the little brook which ran past the schoolhouse and caught minnows to put into it. Or we played catch or knocked flies or grounders with a baseball. Of course we learned much outside of school. Most of us learned about horses, cows and pigs because we had to take care of them.

Hartland Village some twelve miles away had a small

woolen mill and boasted a graded school in the village. At the age of twelve there was an arrangement for me to stay at the home of an aunt in Hartland and go to the grammar school. I did this for one week; but the next Monday morning when my father took me to the station about two miles away, we arrived just in time to see the train pulling out a quarter-mile down the track. I never knew whether or not father missed the train intentionally. Anyhow, with the aid of some neighbors and an unemployed teacher, he organized a private school in the spare room of a neighbor's house.

The next fall three of us from our village went to Maine Central Institute as freshmen after seven years of ungraded school. No certification or examination was involved. M.C.I. was a good academy and gave those of us who were college-bound four years of Latin, two years of French, a year of physics, algebra, geometry and various other things.

I recall one day sitting on the steps of the school building when the principal, Mr. Landman, came out and stopped for a bit of conversation. He said at one stage of our talk, "What do you want to do in life, Turner?"

I replied, "I haven't decided yet what to do, but I want to be among the best at it."

I remember how terribly embarrassed I was when I realized what I had said. Later I realized that most teen-aged boys probably have such ambitions, and I resolved to be sympathetic if, as and when boys expressed them to me.

I entered Bates College in the fall of 1907. I remember conflicting comments the day I appeared on the Bates campus. Because of having deferred tuition, which amounted to $50.00 a year, I went with two of my classmates from M.C.I. to see the president, Dr. Chase. He was most cordial, understanding, and sympathetic. At the end of our discussion he said, "If you young men come back to me at the end of your college course with the same obvious honesty and sincerity, I shall be very happy."

We left his office with the feeling that anyone could see that we were honest and loyal Bates men. We went out to the athletic field to watch football practice, and sat down near the goalposts. The coach came running over and said, "Right off the field, boys. Of course I don't say that you would steal anything, but we've lost a lot of headgears. Sitting here on the field is not allowed."

We wondered who was the better judge of character, the president or the coach.

Because of an intestinal ailment which was probably paratyphoid fever, I came home after three weeks at Bates. It was decided that I should not go back to college that year, and I taught three terms of school.

The fall term was at an ungraded district school in Harmony. Father had retired from medical practice but the family still had a carriage horse. Each school day I put a bag of oats in the buggy; the hired girl put up a lunch for me; I hooked up the horse and drove out to the school.

In mid-winter I taught a ten-week term of "free high school" in the town of Wellington about eight miles to the north. The free high school was for boys and girls who had finished the rural school. They worked on the farm except when the mid-winter snows forced inactivity upon them. In those days the chief excitement of the high school was for the older boys to "carry out" the teacher and throw him into a snowdrift. This gave a few days' vacation until a new teacher could be hired. Fortunately I was spared such an indignity.

The home where I boarded had marvelous food, and it was ten years later before I weighed as much as I did at the end of that term of school. The one subject I had to teach which I had never taken was physical geography.

In the spring I taught the grammar-school class in the village school at St. Albans. The superintendent criticized my lack of discipline, especially with a boy about my size who sat at the back of the room. The next time the superintendent came, it was obvious that the boy was about to start trouble. I walked to the back of the room, leaned over his seat, trying to look as much as possible like a helpful educator giving intellectual assistance to a student. I placed my right hand on the back of his neck and sought a penetration of my thumb and fingers which was far from painless. That solved the behavior problem.

But think of the state of rural schools in those days, when a high school graduate without any preparation for teaching and without any form of certification could teach a rural school, a free high school and a grammar school.

Bates College, to which I returned in the fall of 1908, gave me the usual kind of excellent small college education of those days. It had been founded 44 years earlier and its curriculum offered about half as many courses as it offers today. I had a fifth year of Latin, two years of German, a year of college math, a year of physics, two years of chemistry, and various other subjects. Most importantly I had four years of biology and three years of intercollegiate debating. The first debate was with Massachusetts State College, now the University of Massachusetts. Calvin Coolidge, then Mayor of Northampton, was the Presiding Officer for the debate.

Because of debating credits I could have taken either a Bachelor of Arts or a Bachelor of Science, but my faculty advisor told me that the A.B. was much more distinctive of scholarship than the S.B.

The professor of biology invited me to take a Master's Degree at Harvard and then substitute for him while he was away for a year. I did this before coming to M.I.T., where I found that, with a Master's degree in Biology from Harvard, I needed about a year's study in the mathematical and physical sciences before beginning graduate study in biology and public health.

At M.I.T. my study moved me from biologist to sanitarian and health educator. I began as a graduate student and instructor and remained on the staff for thirty years. These were the days of the growth of the Turner family with my marriage to Naomi Cocke of Austin, Texas, in 1924, the arrival of Mary Frances in 1928 and of Frederick Clair in 1938.

But there was an earlier and somewhat unusual bit of schooling which I ought to tell you about.

This important part of my education between high school and the end of college was the study of interpersonal relations for three "terms." It was called "earning money for college," but it was no less valuable.

The first "term" was the summer after high school when a high-school classmate (Percy T. Clark, who later became a district judge in Ellsworth, Maine) and I sold wire woven brushes from door to door along the Maine coast from Franklin to East Machias.

We each had a suitcase full of sample brushes, and we split our earnings. Our commissions were 40%. Our movements were on foot and mostly confined to villages along the railroad line. Once in going away from the railroad we sent our suitcases by the stage and each took a different road, selling mending tissue to the farm families as we went. The mending tissue of small, rubberlike sheets were in 2″ by 3″ envelopes which sold for 10¢ each and cost us 2¢. It was a very useful product. The purchaser fitted torn cloth back together over a sheet of the mending tissue and applied a hot flatiron. The mending tissue melted and fused the torn pieces of cloth together.

In the spring vacation of my freshman year in college, my college roommate and I sold brushes in Augusta. One day it was so snowy and stormy that calling at homes was quite impossible. With my suitcase of samples I went to the state mental hospital, where a former teacher of mine was a patient. (Not because of my having been her pupil, I trust.) At the door I asked whether a nurse could take me to her, and on the way to her room the nurse promised to take me to the purchasing agent when I finished my visit. The purchasing agent, was quite friendly and gave me an order for about $150 worth of brushes.

The second and third "terms" of my study in interpersonal relations was in making directories. The first one was in Sedgwick, Brooklin, Stonington, Little Deer Island, and

Isle au Haut. In the summer after my sophomore year in college, a classmate and fellow member of the debating team persuaded me to go down on the coast and join him in a directory enterprise.

The other directory was in the summer after our junior year at college, when three of us plus the Turner family horse and buggy made a Somerset County directory in Harmony, Hartland, St. Albans, Palmyra, Pittsfield, Canaan, Athens, Cornville, Detroit, Ripley, and Cambridge.

In making the visit to each family, we told the lady or the man of the house that we were making a directory and asked for information about the family. We recorded the names, the man's occupation, and the married names and location of married children. We also inquired about the previous history of the family in the town, because we included a brief history of each of the towns as well as a map showing the country roads and the location of each house. Our usually cordial receptions were due to the fact that we were dealing with very personal interests of the family, and to the fact that few persons came to the doors of these country homes.

Of course we were taking orders for the book as we went along, but we did not say so. If our technique worked well, the potential customer began to inquire what would be done with these books. We said casually that they would be put in libraries and business firms. When the customer inquired whether he could buy one, we lost no time in asking him to put his name on an order slip, assuring him that we would have one made up for him.

The books were printed in Auburn, Maine. We paid a fixed price per page for 250 copies, plus press costs for copies in excess of that number. The book of 539 pages sold for $1.90. We earned about $300 apiece net for the summer, which went a long way toward college expenses in the early 1900's. I remember many individual experiences, like sleeping in the haymow of a farmer who was First Selectman and to whose home I went to copy the names of town officers.

I remember also the winter visit to Isle au Haut to deliver the books. That scenic island is the top of a mountain sticking up out of the water twenty miles from the mainland. A tremendous northeast storm drove waves against the rocks, sending the water fifty feet into the air.

The most valuable part of the directory business was learning to understand people.

# 9

## I REMEMBER A GREAT TEACHER

It was on a clear, crisp Saturday morning in the spring of 1913 that I first met Professor William Thompson Sedgwick. I remember my excitement as I made my way along the streets of Boston's Back Bay, past the Boston Public Library and the Phillips Brooks Church to the brick building in Trinity Place which housed the Department of Biology and Public Health of M.I.T. Albert Buck, who had graduated with me at Bates College the previous June, was studying in Sedgwick's department and initiated an appointment for me.

Albert met me at the door and took me up a flight of stairs to a rather small library reading room-waiting room, presided over by Professor Sedgwick's secretary, whom I later came to know as Miss Esterbrook. It was she who took me to Professor Sedgwick's office, which was as small for an office as the main room was for a library. Books and files of papers filled the shelves, which ran to the ceiling, and spilled over onto the floor and a couple of extra chairs.

Professor Sedgwick was seated at his desk. His cordial smile and greeting immediately dispelled my nervousness.

"Your classmate told me you are studying biology, Mr. Turner. What do you want to do with your life?" he said.

"I would like to teach," I replied.

"Really? I almost never have a student who wants to teach," was his rejoinder. "You will never make much money at that, you know. But you won't starve. You might get a job like mine, do a little consultation, and write a book or two."

That was what I remember best of the conversation, which

lasted a few minutes and ended with his advice that I should keep in touch with him if I was interested in the kinds of things his department was doing.

I left his office walking on air. Nobody had ever suggested such professional possibilities. Even if they were only half true, life was much brighter than it had seemed to me in recent months—when, after embarking upon the quest for a Master's degree at Harvard six weeks after the fall semester had begun, I had been working long days, six and a half days a week.

The next fall I went to Bates to take the place of the head of the Biology Department while he was on sabbatical leave for a year. My year's salary was $1,000. In a letter to Professor Sedgwick on January 5, 1914, I said, "After investigating the courses in bacteriology offered by various institutions, I have become thoroughly convinced that I wish to do my work at Massachusetts Institute of Technology. I am therefore coming to Tech next fall to study as long as my finances will allow, even if it be for but one semester."

A return letter from Professor Sedgwick said, "We are all pleased to think that you may like to come and work with us next fall, and I wish to do my best to make it possible for you to spend the whole year. We shall certainly need assistance next year, and if you could help us with some of our classes, I am very sure that we shall be able to free you from tuition fees."

In March I received a letter from Professor Sedgwick offering me a job as biologist to work with a chemist in the study of the self-purification processes of a stream which had been polluted with the treated sewage of the City of Brockton. This work, which began July 1, 1914, marked the commencement of a close contact with Professor Sedgwick which continued until his death.

His ability to expect the best of his students was an important quality of Professor Sedgwick in producing graduates like E. O. Jordan, 1888, who became Professor of Bacteriology at the University of Chicago and the author of the first widely used textbook in general bacteriology; George C. Whipple, 1889, later Professor of Sanitary Engineering at Harvard; C. E.-A. Winslow, 1898, who established the public health program at Yale University; Selskar M. Gunn, 1905, who later became director of the Rockefeller Institute in Paris; and many other men and women of distinction. I realized this trait and vowed to follow his example; but, frankly, I found it very difficult to do. Even with the full realization that one's students tend to live up to great expectation and live down to lesser expectation, those of us who are more ordinary than Sedgwick tend to compare student abilities and imply limitations.

Professor Sedgwick also had the ability to fix the eyes of his "boys" (as he and Mrs. Sedgwick called his students) on a distant star and at the same time to point out the stumbling-block just ahead. I remember the day he called me to his office and said, "There is a job as assistant to Professor Rosenau, and I think, if you agree, you should apply for it. But I have a suggestion for you. You are inclined to be too passive and wait for the other person to carry the conversation. When you go to Professor Rosenau's office, lean forward in your seat and say, 'Professor Rosenau, I am greatly interested in this job and I think I can do it well.' "

I did as Professor Sedgwick advised. Professor Rosenau seemed surprised, even startled; but his immediate reaction was, "By jove, I believe you would do well. You can have the job."

Actually, developments at Tech were such that I did not take the post; but this diagnosis and prescription for a personality defect was very helpful, even though perhaps a single prescription could not effect a permanent cure for a deep-seated malady.

Significant also was Professor Sedgwick's kindliness. He was always helping us in the most kindly manner with the details of our activities, our planning, and our oral or written statements. When the two-year study of stream-purification was finished I prepared the report for publication. It went directly to the typesetter, probably because Professor Sedgwick was too busy at the moment to read the manuscript. He did read the proof sheets, and it was difficult to find the type under his blue-pencil marks when he had finished. He gave back the pages to me with a most friendly comment that this kind of copy needs special care in preparation and that "it will be cheapest to have a fresh copy made and let the printer start all over again."

One day the switchboard operator at Tech referred to me a telephone call from a woman who wanted some advice about the drain from her kitchen sink. I happened to mention this to Professor Sedgwick, and his comment was, "I'm glad you helped her. Here we do anything for anybody, do it well, and do it for nothing."

Professor Sedgwick was not only a great teacher, he was one of the most distinguished pioneers in public health. His most important scientific achievements are reflected in a biography by three of his former students, published by the Yale University Press in 1924 *(William Thompson Sedgwick —a Pioneer in Public Health,* by E. O. Jordan, G. C. Whipple and C. E.-A. Winslow, with an introduction by Mary K. Sedgwick). This book lists 124 scientific publications.

Sedgwick was born in West Hartford, Connecticut, on December 29, 1855. He took his Bachelor's Degree at the Sheffield Scientific School of Yale in 1877 and his Ph.D. in the Biological Sciences at Johns Hopkins in 1881. He was married to Mary K. Rice on December 29 of that year and came to M.I.T. as an Associate Professor in 1883, where he later became Professor and Head of the Department of Biology and Public Health.

The first bacteriological culture media to come to this country from Europe were brought to Professor Sedgwick by Dr. Nichols in 1886. The first water and sewage bacteriology to be undertaken in America was begun in Professor Sedgwick's laboratory in 1887. The work of Professor Sedgwick and Dr. Drown of the M.I.T. for the State Department of Health laid the foundation for our most important processes of sewage purification. Professor Sedgwick was a pioneer epidemiologist in his study of the typhoid fever epidemics along the Merrimac River in the early 1890's. The first course in epidemiology was offered at M.I.T.

The year I came to Tech (1914) Professor Sedgwick was about to enter upon the presidency of the American Public Health Association, and Professor Gunn in his department was editor of the Association's journal. In a letter to me April 12, 1919, he mentions an interesting professional relationship in saying, "You will be interested to know that I have been commissioned 'Directing Sanitary Engineer' with the Grade of Assistant Surgeon General in the Reserve of the U.S. Public Health Service."

Professor Sedgwick's pioneering developments in establishing the Department of Biology and Public Health at Tech and as Chairman of the Harvard-M.I.T. School of Public Health, stamp him as one of the greatest pioneer educators in the public health field.

# 10

## THE SELF-PURIFICATION OF STREAMS

The letter from the Department of Biology and Public Health at M.I.T. in which Professor Sedgwick offered me a job as the biologist in studying the self-purification of streams came to me at Bates College in March, 1914. I came to Boston on July 1 and met Mr. Ralph Bates, who was to work with me as a chemist. He had just graduated from Tech in Course XI (Sanitary Engineering). We proceeded to Brockton and arranged to board with a family near the sewage filtration works. Together we set up a laboratory for chemical, bacteriological and biological studies in the testing laboratory of the sewage purification plant.

The situation we were to study was most interesting. Up to that time there had been no intensive investigation of what takes place biologically when the partially purified sewage effluent from a city is discharged into a river. The chemical steps by which nitrogenous substances are transformed into nitrates were well understood, as well as the processes of dilution, sedimentation and bacterial action; but there had never been a detailed study of the biology of the self-purification of streams.

The Sanitary Research Laboratory of M.I.T. had issued nine volumes of studies dealing mainly with the chemical and bacteriological processes of sewage purification. Robert Spurr Weston, a distinguished sanitary engineer, was a lecturer in Professor Sedgwick's department, and it was he who proposed a study of what happens *biologically* in stream-purification. The site chosen was the Coweeset Stream before and after receiving the sandbed effluent from the sewage purification plant of the City of Brockton, a city of about 64,000 people. The 2,000,000-gallon daily effluent from the several one-acre sandbed filters was a liquid low in color but high in various nitrogen compounds. It was thrown into a stream of about 5,000,000 gallons' daily flow.

The study continued for two years and was published as Volume 10 of the Sanitary Research Laboratory Reports. It was entitled, *Study on the Digestion of a Sewage-Filter Effluent by a Small and Otherwise Unpolluted Stream.* Mr. Bates spent his full time on the project. I worked full time during the two summers, but in the school year I came to Boston four mornings a week to attend classes in the public health courses I was taking.

Brockton is about 21 miles from Boston, and at that time train service exactly fitted my needs. I left Brockton at 8:16 in the morning and in returning I left the Back Bay Station in Boston, which was only a block from the M.I.T. building which housed the Department of Biology and Public Health, at 12:05.

My function was to determine which species of plants and animals (microscopic and macroscopic) were in the stream at different points and at different times of year. We established sampling stations, one above the point where the sewage effluent came in, and eight below that point. Stations 2 to 6 were located at short distances below the point of pollution; station 7 was two miles and station 8 was 3½ miles below the sewage plant. Samples from the upper stations we collected on foot. Samples for the two lower stations were collected on bicycles, each having a rack for bottles back of the seat. I remember being thrown clean off the loaded bike at different times when the wheels slid into a rut.

Our sampling and testing was fairly extensive. We made weekly physical tests to determine stream turbidity, temperature and color; and chemical tests of total nitrogen, free ammonia, albuminoid ammonia, carbon dioxide, nitrites and nitrates. We also measured dissolved oxygen and oxygen consumed in the water samples.

Our biological samples were run through a Sedgwick-Rafter filter, a device previously developed by Professor Sedgwick and one of his students for collecting and studying microscopic organisms from the water of city reservoirs. This device is a glass tube about two feet in length and 2½ inches in diameter, reduced at the bottom to a diameter of less than an inch. Clean sand is put in the tube, held in place by a rubber stopper with holes in it. A piece of clean bolting-cloth prevents the sand from going through the stopper. Known volumes of water are filtered through the device until the water volume has been reduced to five cubic centimeters. This water and the organisms contained are washed off from the sand and studied under the microscope.

I knew the different major groups of plants and animals, of course, but I remember well my feelings of frustration when I found in the samples dozens of species of protozoa, rotifers, microscopic crustacea, diatoms, algae, and other plants and animals which I had never seen before.

The study of our samples and the pursuit of sanitary engineering literature soon made me a fresh-water biologist of sorts and also made me somewhat conversant with the major problems of waste disposal. When I started the job it was so frustrating as to be distasteful, although many of the individual plants and animals were beautiful and had fascinating life histories. At the end of the two-year study I had a list of over thirty research problems which I would have greatly enjoyed pursuing. The more one knows about a subject, the more interesting it becomes, and almost any field can become a hobby when one knows enough about it.

You will have limited interest in the detailed findings of this study, which showed the sequence of changes taking place in the polluted stream, the organisms involved, and the predilection of different species of plants and animals for different conditions. Chemical changes and biological activities were most rapid in the high temperatures of summer. Some organisms were plentiful at one season and absent or nearly absent at other seasons. For example a mold *(Lep-*

*tomitus)* which grew into a mat thicker than that of bread mold, appeared each fall as the weather became cold, first at the outlet of the drains from the filters. Later it became so plentiful as to form a mat over the whole bottom of the stream. It disappeared when the warm weather of spring came. The disappearance started at the farthest point downstream. We used to say it came out of the drains in the fall and went back into the drains in the spring.

In general this sequence of events occurred. There were few plants or animals of any kind in the clear water of the stream above the point where the pollution occurred. For the first few hundred yards below that point the bacterial content of the water was tremendous. Then the numbers of organisms that feed on bacteria reached a great height. These were mainly ciliate protozoa and rotifera. Microscopic crustacea were abundant. A couple of miles below the source of pollution we found trout and other fish. The biological story presented a clear picture of the translation of dissolved proteins into fishmeat. At the time of the spring floods the Coweeset overflowed its banks a half-mile below the sewage plant, forming a lake 150 yards wide, which became filled with green algae carrying on their oxygen-producing processes.

This study showed the nature, intensity and possibilities of the biological processes in the self-purification of streams. Today engineers use the biological processes of sewage purification by constructing lagoons of shallow water into which sewage or sewage-filter effluents are discharged.

# 11

## A.P.H.A.

One of the best places to look for the development of a profession is in the history of its professional association. The American Public Health Association is 100 years old this year (1972); but when I came to M.I.T. in 1914 the possibility of joining this still relatively new profession was stimulating and exciting. The great growth of the association has been since then. In 1916 its membership was 1,647, but it had doubled since 1910. Its seven sections were Public Health Administration, Laboratory, Sociology, Industrial Hygiene, Sanitary Engineering, Vital Statistics, and Food. Today (1972) its membership is approximately 22,000. It has 20 sections and 55 affiliated associations and regional branches.

Another way to picture the youth of the public health profession is to point out that my generation studied public health under leaders who were already young men while Louis Pasteur (1822-1895) was alive and carrying on those fundamental discoveries of communicable diseases which opened the door to preventive medicine and today's health programs. These were men like William T. Sedgwick (1855-1921) at M.I.T.; William H. Welch (1850-1934) of Johns Hopkins University; Victor C. Vaughan (1851-1929) at the University of Michigan; George C. Whipple (1866-1924), a pioneer in Sanitary Engineering at Harvard; and Edwin O. Jordan (1866-1936), the bacteriologist at the University of Chicago.

Men and women in my age group were already in college (1911) when the association established its journal, the

*American Journal of Public Health.* Between 1910 and 1970 the population of the United States a little more than doubled, but the membership of the A.P.H.A. increased over 25-fold. In 1922 many of us became charter fellows of the newly established fellowship classification in A.P.H.A. which was offered to "those who had attained a certain degree of eminence in the field."

My first participation in an A.P.H.A. meeting was at Rochester, New York, in the fall of 1915. My last paper was 57 years later (1972) at the 100th Anniversary meeting in Atlantic City. At the Rochester meeting I of course was not in a position to present a paper. But it was the second year of the Brockton study; and Professor Sedgwick was so good as to open the way for me to participate in a discussion of the Sanitary Engineering Section. I remember that he said to the chairman of the meeting that "We at M.I.T. are studying stream-purification. Mr. Turner, who is in charge of the study, is present, and I would like him to tell us the nature of his investigation."

Like the many moderately active members of the association, I had a variety of activities in A.P.H.A. between 1915 and 1972. They included publication of many papers and reports; membership on the Governing Council in 1928-30, 1942 and 1957-58; membership on the Executive Board in 1928-29 and 1933-35; Secretaryship of the Child Hygiene Section 1923-26; and Chairmanship of the Health Education Section in 1939.

My most interesting activity in A.P.H.A. had to do with professional education in public health. In 1919 some of us at M.I.T. discussed the need for an agreement as to what professional education should be required. We took up the question with the president of the association and the topic was put on the list of considerations to come before the executive board. An interesting discussion took place at the board meeting, where it was pointed out that Professor Winslow had earlier suggested steps in this direction. It was decided to have such a committee; and the president appointed a Committee of Sixteen with Professor Winslow as chairman and myself as secretary. The other members of the committee were Dr. A. C. Abbott, Dr. Mark Boyd, Dr. L. D. Bristol, Dr. W. H. Brown, Dr. J. C. Geiger, Mr. Samuel A. Greeley, Professor E. O. Jordan, Dr. Arthur I. Kendall, Dr. R. T. Legge, Dr. W. H. Park, Professor M. J. Rosenau, Professor W. T. Sedgwick, Dr. Victor Vaughan and Dr. William H. Welch.

Our first report was published in the April 1921 issue of the *American Journal of Public Health;* and it reported quite completely upon what degrees and certificates in public health were granted by universities in the United States and Canada. Eight different degrees, certificates or diplomas were offered in 25 universities.

I continued as Secretary through 1923 and took over the Chairmanship in 1924. This beginning led to some three decades of work on this committee or upon the Sub-Committee on the Professional Education of Community Health Educators. These committees produced a long series of reports having much to do in shaping the educational requirements for public health degrees.

## 12

# ADVENTURES IN LEGISLATION AND SANITATION

My first adventure in promoting public health action came in the winter of 1916-17. It began at a meeting of the Boston Alumni of Bates College. Governor Carl Milliken of Maine was, like myself, a Bates graduate, and I had a chance to talk with him at the mid-winter Boston Bates reunion. I asked the governor when Maine would establish a more effective state health department. He said that the State Medical Society was supporting a bill in the legislature; and he asked why, since I was still a legal resident of Maine, I should not come down to lobby for the bill. I reported this conversation to Professor Sedgwick, who suggested immediately that he would give me a few weeks' leave from M.I.T. to go to Augusta. I went to Maine and contacted Dr. Sylvester Judd Beach, who was Chairman of the State Medical Society Legislative Committee.

It was fortunate that I was still a legal citizen of Maine, because every legislator I approached asked me why someone should come to Augusta from Massachusetts to influence legislation. The answer that I was a voting citizen of Maine was, in every case, the perfect reply.

Actually, the bill originally introduced by the Medical Society placed so much power in the hands of the Commissioner of Health as to make the plan seem dangerous. Dr. Beach agreed that this was the case; and we decided to substitute for the original bill a plan which was essentially that recently adopted by both Massachusetts and New York, providing for a State Commissioner of Health and a State Public Health Council.

Conferences with the members of the Public Health Committee of the Legislature involved considerable time discussing the situation in detail, as did conferences with the committee chairman, Dr. Phillips, a general practitioner in Maine who was deeply interested in public health. He agreed with the idea of substituting a bill similar to the new law in Massachusetts but adapted to the State of Maine. The legislators were going to Portland for a special meeting. On the train between Lewiston and Portland, Dr. Phillips, two other members of his committee, and I agreed on the changes needed in the Massachusetts bill. Dr. Beach resided in Portland, and that evening I reported to him the progress to date, telling him that we were now assured that the Public Health Committee would report favorably upon the bill.

Professor Sedgwick was very helpful through correspondence with key men in the legislature. On March 19 he wrote the following letter to the Public Health Committee:

Mar. 19, 1917

The Public Health Committee,
State House
Augusta, Maine

Gentlemen:

I understand from my associate, Professor Turner, that there is a good chance that the State of Maine may fall into line with New York and Massachusetts in substituting for a Board of Health a Commissioner of Health.

Allow me to say that in Massachusetts the new plan which was inaugurated under Governor Walsh has been carried out in a thoroughly non-partisan manner, and with increased efficiency and improved service in every respect.

I am myself a member of the Public Health Council of the State Department of Massachusetts, and also a Member of the Advisory Board, Hygienic Laboratory,

U.S. Public Health Service, and I beg leave to advise and urge upon you most respectfully the substitution of the new plan for the old.

The fact is that the full time of a highly trained man is now needed and that the natural check upon such a person furnished by the Public Health Council, together with the representation of different sections of the State, is a combination yielding high efficiency with the essentials of Democracy.

May I take the liberty of adding that I am a propertyholder as a summer resident of the Town of Mt. Desert, Maine, and that down that way we are all keenly interested in the good work already done by the Maine Board, and in aiding in every possible way in improving this work.

Public Health today is a term to conjure with, and such phrases as infant mortality, rural sanitation, industrial hygiene and the control of infectious diseases, are attracting public attention and public interest on every hand. I honestly believe that if the State of Maine wishes to keep up with the procession it should join the new movement and take its place along with Massachusetts and New York, which are leaders in it.

Very respectfully yours,
/s/ W. T. Sedgwick
Professor of Biology and Public Health,
and Chairman, School for Health Officers,
Harvard University and Massachusetts
Institute of Technology

On March 21 he wrote to the Chairman of the Committee, Dr. Phillips, as follows:

March 21, 1917

Dear Dr. Phillips:

My associate, Mr. Turner, whom you have probably met by this time, comes from Maine and is deeply interested in the improvement of your State Board of Health.

Mr. Turner is not looking for a job for himself, for we propose to keep him right here at the Tech. But he is a conscientious, high-toned, progressive man, and wants to see his native state come forward and do what it ought to do for public health.

I am on the Public Health Council of the Massachusetts State Dept. of Health, and have long been familiar both with the old Board and the new, and I can say to you without any hesitation that the New York-Massachusetts plan works infinitely better than the old State Board of Health plan and need not cost much more.

I greatly hope that you will be good to Mr. Turner and that you will, if consonant with your own convictions, work hard for the adoption in the State of Maine of the New York-Massachusetts plan, in which I heartily believe.

With kindest regards,

Sincerely yours,
/s/ W. T. Sedgwick

Dr. J. D. Phillips,
Committee on Public Health,
State House, Augusta, Maine

Because Maine is a famous vacation state, legislators are interested in the wishes of their summer residents as well as in the opinions of their full-time citizens. The following letter from President Eliot of Harvard University is typical of a very appreciable number of letters which Professor Sedgwick arranged to have sent to the Public Health Committee:

Cambridge, Mass.
22 March, 1917

Dear Sir:

As I have been a property holder at Mount Desert,

Maine, and a summer resident there for many years, I venture to urge upon you the importance of improving by public legislation the organization of the State Board of Health of Maine.

The State Board of Health of Massachusetts led the country for more than twenty years as regards organization and work. Lately New York adopted an organization superior to that of Massachusetts; and this better organization Massachusetts has adopted.

It is certain that Maine might wisely adopt the Massachusetts-New York organization for promoting the health of the State. The State has no higher function than that of preserving and promoting the health and vigor of its people.

Sincerely yours,
/s/ Charles W. Eliot
President

To Chairman of the Maine
Public Health Committee

Other letters came from such men as Selskar M. Gunn, the editor of the *American Journal of Public Health,* and Lee K. Frankel, Third Vice-President of the Metropolitan Life Insurance Company.

It was pleasant contacting key legislators suggested to me by Dr. Phillips and discussing the bill with them. I also went to Bowdoin College to see Professor Marshall Cram, chairman of the existing State Board of Health, who was most courteous and who wrote me a nice letter on March 27 saying that he would not stand in the way of this bill and that he believed the other members of the present board would not.

An important Christian Science practitioner opposed the bill, but his main concern was the possible danger that the law might restrict the forms of practice in the cure of disease. He withdrew his vigorous opposition when we very properly inserted in the bill a statement indicating that nothing in this bill should interfere with the right of the individual to choose the methods of treatment of his choice.

The excitement involved is reflected in the following letter from Dr. Beach under date of April Sixth:

Apr. 6, 1917

Mr. C. E. Turner,
M.I.T., Cambridge, Mass.

My dear Mr. Turner:

The bill had an uneventful career up to yesterday when it had the scare of its life. It got passed to be engrossed as you know, and some economist whose name I forget got up and said that he felt that in the present national tumult we ought not to spend any more money and moved that it be postponed indefinitely. Somebody else speaking for the present board said that he felt it was unnecessary and the motion to postpone indefinitely was lost by a vote of 41 to 43. It was then passed to be enacted. I suppose if anyone is really out for it, he can stall it any time before it is passed. As I understand it, it has yet to be finally passed.

Cordially yours,
/s/ S. J. Beach

The bill did go through, and Dr. L. D. Bristol, a physician with graduate training in public health at Harvard, was appointed Commissioner of Health in the new department. It did not seem feasible to me to accept an offered long-term appointment in Maine, but I did accept on appointment to make a sanitary survey in the summer of 1917 covering summer resorts, hotels, lumber camps, and trains.

This survey was a thoroughly delightful experience personally, in addition to giving me a chance to apply standards of sanitation and an opportunity to see vacation resorts of the greatest interest. I remember especially a week visiting hotels in the lake region, when I borrowed a canoe each day after supper and stayed out on the lake through the setting of the sun and establishing of moonlight.

The existence of a single case of typhoid fever in a lumber camp caused the Commissioner of Health to send me into the deep Maine woods to inspect lumber-camp sanitation. This gave me a chance to see the nature of lumbering operations and to work with the progressive American Thread Company in the sanitation of their industry.

The studying of sanitation on passenger trains was not extensive, as the number of trains on the Maine Central Railroad and the Bangor and Aroostook Railroad was rather limited.

Reports on these activities appeared in the following publications, reprints of which are in the Turner Collection at the A. O. Deweese Memorial Library of the American School Health Association at Kent, Ohio:

> "Rules and Regulations of the State Department of Health Governing the Sanitary Conditions of Hotels"; "Cooperation between Hotels and State Department of Health in Maine"; "A Sanitary Reconnaissance of Hotels, Passenger Trains and Lumber Camps in the State of Maine"; "Hotel Inspection in the State of Maine"; "Work in the Maine Woods"; "Health and Personal Comfort Assured in American Thread Co. Lumber Camps"; "Living Conditions in the Maine Woods."

## 13

## WORLD WAR I AND THE GREAT PANDEMIC

My participation in World War I was as a Sanitary Engineer, First Lieutenant Grade, in the U.S. Public Health Service. (The Public Health Service was made a part of the armed services later in the war. However, my major's commission in the U.S. Army Sanitary Corps came after the end of the war.) My assignment was to the Emergency Fleet Corporation under Colonel Philip Doane, and involved the health supervision of shipyards in Connecticut, Massachusetts, New Hampshire and Maine. The yards in question employed a total of about 25,000 men, and varied in size from yards constructing wooden ships and having only 150 men to the Foreriver Shipyard of the Bethlehem Steel Corp. in Quincy, Mass., which employed about 15,000 men and had as its Assistant Works Manager Mr. Joseph Kennedy, the father of President John Kennedy.

Officers like myself were assigned to districts along the Atlantic, Gulf and Pacific coasts. We were told privately that the pressure for ships was so great that we must work with the shipyards through cooperation rather than through rigid commands which would slow up ship production. Our routine work involved supervision over general sanitation, food production, housing, and first-aid facilities.

The one tremendously exciting development was the influenza pandemic in the fall of 1918. This was one of the greatest pandemics of all time. Between September and December 1918, 500,000 Americans perished from influenza and nearly 20,000,000 persons had the disease. The devastations of the disease in other parts of the world were comparable to those in North America, producing a morbidity and mortality greater than had ever been seen in such a short period of time.

The earliest recorded cases in the United States arrived on an army transport late in the month of August. These few typical cases were taken to the Chelsea Naval Hospital. Other cases were soon reported from among the 5,000 sailors then on duty at Commonwealth Pier, about half of whom were quartered among the civil population of Greater Boston. The presence of the disease was not generally known, however, nor was its seriousness realized, until about the second week in September, when an emergency hospital was established for the men in the training division of the U.S. Shipping Board.

Public health activities in the shipbuilding industry involved programs to keep morbidity and mortality at the lowest possible level (C. E. Turner, "Organizing an Industry to Combat Influenza," *Journal of Industrial Hygiene,* Vol. I, May 1919–June 1920).

The procedural steps in my district were as follows:

1. The general manager of each plant was warned by telephone or telegram of the danger which threatened his organization. That communication was followed by a confirming letter outlining the situation and the steps needed for disease control.

2. The industrial physician in each plant was given all the available facts regarding the nature of the disease, its treatment, the clinical appearance of the cases already under treatment in Boston, and the advisability of prompt isolation and bedside precautions.

3. A special cooperating organization was created in each yard consisting of: (a) the physician and nurse at the first-aid rooms; (b) an assistant to the physician, where necessary, who attended to non-medical details; and (c) the foremen in the yard, who were instructed by means of printed directions prepared by the sanitary engineer and distributed with the added authority of the yard management. These instruc-

tions outlined the symptoms of the disease and stated the necessity of immediately sending all men with such symptoms to the plant physician or nurse. Workmen who had been excluded because of the disease were required to check with the physician's office before going back on the job.

4. The cooperation of the local, state and federal public health agencies was secured, and it was arranged that they should receive prompt reports of all cases occurring in the industry.

5. Posters or signs prepared at the yard warning against special dangers of infection were posted near the gates where employees entered and left. The following copy was used for most of these posters:

> IF YOU HAVE COLD OR GRIPPE REPORT TO DOCTOR IMMEDIATELY.
> BEWARE OF ANY MEN COUGHING OR SNEEZING.
> WHEN YOU COUGH COVER MOUTH WITH HAND.
> AVOID PUBLIC GATHERINGS . . . THEATRES . . . DANCES, ETC.
> DO NOT SPIT ON MATERIAL THAT MUST BE HANDLED.
> GET GOOD FOOD AND ENOUGH SLEEP.

6. Hospital and treatment facilities were arranged in advance of the actual appearance of cases. In most instances some barrack or other building on the shipyard property was transformed into an emergency hospital.

7. The use of common drinking cups was immediately discontinued in all yards and individual paper drinking cups with special sanitary distributing buckets were supplied.

8. The complete scalding of all dishes in restaurants, hotels and barracks was required.

9. Special supervision over food handlers was instituted with examinations twice daily, in order that no person han-

dling food for shipyard workers should continue work with the slightest symptoms of the disease.

10. Educational pamphlets upon the subject of influenza were distributed to men in all yards.

11. Daily reports from each yard were received at the Boston office, indicating the number of cases appearing at the yard hospital during the preceding 24 hours.

12. Follow-up posters warning against the dangers of sequelae were posted in all yards.

It was, of course, difficult to keep in sufficiently close touch with the eleven different shipyards to see that suitable programs were established and operated. There was constant pressure. For example, one day upon returning to the Boston office at about 6 P.M. I found a letter from the supervisor of the district, accompanied by copy of a telegram from the Washington office to a shipyard between Dover and Portsmouth, N. H., saying in effect that Sanitary Engineer Turner had earlier reported unsanitary crowding in the sleeping quarters of their dormitory and instructed the shipyard to place correction of the situation under my supervision. I was requested to take the late evening train to Portsmouth where I could get a few hours' sleep in the first-aid room at a Portsmouth plant, and to report to the manager of the other shipyard at 8 o'clock in the morning.

In general the established program was reasonably successful. No yard had more than 10% of the working force affected. We believed that the intense supervision over dining rooms and food handlers, as well as the prompt isolation of workmen showing symptoms, was especially important. Mortality records from 24,350 men showed 85 deaths between September 15 and March 1, which were directly attributed to influenza. This was a death rate of 3.49 per thousand. In no yard was the death rate in excess of 5 per thousand. The U.S. Public Health Service reports for August 15, 1919 showed a death rate for the cities east of the Appalachian Mountains of 5.6 per thousand population for the same period.

One other activity in the shipyard experience may interest you. There were a few months after the armistice was signed before the health program in shipyards was concluded. Our larger shipyards had employee safety committees in the various work departments. We arranged for these committees to become "Safety *and Health* Committees," and found that interest and accomplishment in health improvement was readily possible with these groups.

# 14

# THE FIRST PROGRAM OF STUDY IN HEALTH EDUCATION AT A SCHOOL OF PUBLIC HEALTH

In the Presidential Address before the Society for Public Health Education in October 1971 Scott Simonds said, "The profession is fifty years old, using the start of professional preparation in 1921 as the founding date." The "professional preparation" to which he referred was the program of study in health education established in the Harvard-M.I.T. School of Public Health in the school year 1921-22 and built around the new course in health education which we were introducing at M.I.T. How did this come about?

Professor Sedgwick had an interesting practice of looking for current and future needs in the expanding field of public health, as illustrated in the following episode:

One day soon after my return from service in World War I (1919) he called me into his office and said, "Mr. Turner, I'd like you to come back in two weeks and tell me what desirable activities in public health we are not doing at all or only inadequately, and what might be done in that area."

Two weeks later I went back to him to say that I believed we should help the public to take greater and more intelligent responsibility in the care of its own health. We discussed possibilities. Professor Sedgwick said, "Let's go ahead. The place to start should be the public schools, because everyone goes to school."

Arrangements were made for me to experiment in a school in Somerville. These experiments, which were followed by more extensive studies in the City of Malden, led to the suggestion that we should establish a program of study in the

School of Public Health for students who wished to equip themselves for work in this field. Professor Sedgwick asked me to suggest such a program of study.

On Saturday, January 25, 1921, I brought such a proposed plan to his office. We discussed the suggestions, which met with his cordial approval. In the midst of our discussion, Professor C. E.-A. Winslow came to see Professor Sedgwick.

"Come in, Charlie," said Professor Sedgwick. "I'm just approving a plan of Mr. Turner's to accept some graduate students next fall to prepare themselves for the kind of work in health education with which we have been experimenting."

We discussed plans a bit and Professor Winslow said, "This is a good idea. Go ahead with it, and I think in two or three years we can do this sort of thing at Yale."

The next day, Sunday, January 26, 1921, Professor Sedgwick came home from an evening committee meeting. He retired to his bedroom. Mrs. Sedgwick, who was sitting in the living room, heard him fall and he never spoke again. He was dead from cerebral hemorrhage.

His last official act was the approval of instruction in health education at M.I.T. It was characteristic of the man that this last activity, like so many of his earlier ones, dealt with a new development. He had earlier introduced public health into the Department of Biology at M.I.T. No other pioneer in public health of his generation could have been more sympathetic to health education as a new idea.

Professor Winslow's visit to Professor Sedgwick that Saturday morning was a happy coincidence. Professor Prescott, who became Head of the Department of Biology and Public Health following the death of Professor Sedgwick, approved the program, and in 1921-22 the first course in health education ever offered in a School of Public Health was given at M.I.T., which was then cooperating in the Harvard-M.I.T. School of Public Health.

That was the last year of the Harvard-M.I.T. School. The next year the Harvard School of Public Health was formed, but each year for over twenty years some students from that school came to Tech for work in health education until Harvard established its own program in that field.

Experimentation in health education had begun promptly after Professor Sedgwick first approved the idea. It was possible to arrange at the West School in the City of Somerville for me to meet twice a week with a fourth-grade class and a fifth-grade class. These meetings were the periods of the health course. We began monthly weighing of children to interest them in growth, and I had individual health-habit conferences with children who were not growing well. The sessions with the children were most pleasant for me and apparently also for them. It was particularly pleasing as we came toward the end of the school year to have some of the parents say that they would miss the health program during the vacation because it aided so much in promoting hygienic living. The wife of a physician said she liked the health program and that her boy would do some things for the teacher that he would not do for his own father.

The later studies in Malden continued over a ten-year period in three experimental schools, with three similar control schools being used as a check on various developments. The classroom activities in the Malden studies were under my general direction but were immediately in the hands of Miss Georgie B. Collins, a former teacher of one of the classes in Somerville with which the experimentation had begun.

The following experience in planning this study reflected both the limitation of funds and our belief in what we were undertaking. The Superintendent of Schools in Malden agreed to pay Miss Collins' salary, and she naturally inquired about her contract.

"You do not get any contract," said Superintendent Marshall. "This plan looks good, but if it should backfire I want to be free to stop it immediately and not continue it until the end of the school year." I assured him that I felt the same way and that we would find something for Miss Collins to do at M.I.T. if the experimentation was not successful.

The Malden studies showed us many desirable and some undesirable procedures. They led to the abandonment nationally of unsound practices with regard to "underweight children." They showed that desirable improvement could be produced in habits of nutrition, exercise, rest and other phases of healthful living, and they gave us interesting information with regard to the significance of intermittency in growth. The methods we developed became the basis of a widely used series of textbooks from grades 3 to 9 inclusive. Our M.I.T. instruction at the graduate level in the preparation of health educators included expanding activities in health education methods for the adult community as well as activities in school health education.

# 15

# THE FIRST HEALTH TEACHING FILMS

One morning in 1919, not long after we had begun to experiment with health education in schools, Professor Sedgwick sent his secretary to ask me to come to his office to meet Dr. Edwin O. Jordan, Professor of Bacteriology at the University of Chicago.

When introductions were over, Professor Sedgwick asked Dr. Jordan to explain a situation the two of them had been discussing. It seemed that there had been organized in Chicago a society for visual education. The president was Harley Clarke, a public-spirited utility administrator. The secretary was Forest Ray Moulton, Professor of Mathematics at the University of Chicago, who later became the editor of *Science*.

A public health committee had been formed consisting of Professor Jordan, Professor Victor Vaughan of the University of Michigan, Professor William Welsh of Johns Hopkins, and Dr. Hans Zinsser of the Rockefeller Foundation. Professor Jordan said that the committee was so distinguished and so busy that no one in the group had any time to give to the planning of motion pictures. Professor Sedgwick had pointed out that I was interested in teaching health in the public schools, and he suggested that I might become the Secretary of the committee. This arrangement was made.

Letters from me to the members of the committee made some suggestions and asked for comments and proposals. Approval and comments were received promptly from all of the members of the committee except Dr. Welsh. Not hearing from him was disappointing because his discovery of the

*Bacillus Welchii* and his other researches had made him one of the world's best-known men in public health. Finally, however, a letter did come. It was in longhand and reflected real enthusiasm. Not being satisfied with correspondence alone, he invited me to come to Baltimore for dinner with him at the Maryland Club, and to spend the evening discussing possibilities. This visit with Dr. Welsh in the late years of his distinguished career supplied one of my most cherished memories.

The Society for Visual Education was making films in the various basic school subjects. Dr. Wallace Atwood, a distinguished geographer and a Professor at Harvard, who later became President of Clark University, was making films in geography. He had the remarkable ability of drawing on the blackboard with both hands at once, and the creation of maps in this way provided one interesting feature of the geography films.

The society arranged for animated photography, but most of the direct photography was done under my direction in Boston. We found school-age children to be natural actors. With them we could decide what we wanted to show and go ahead at once to film the action. Adults needed at least two or three rehearsals for each activity.

Our first two films dealt with "The Self-Purification of Streams," telling the story of our recent research in Brockton, and with "Diphtheria," telling mainly the story of how diphtheria antitoxin is produced. Over the next several years, with some assistance in writing scenarios, we continued film-making as a special or incidental activity. A list of these films follows:

*Circulatory Control*
*Good Foods: A Drink of Water*
*Clean Clothes*
*First Aid—Care of Minor Wounds*
*Circulation*
*Care of the Teeth*

*The Skin*
*Home Nursing: Routine Procedures*
*Diphtheria*
*Microorganisms*
*Bacteria*
*Posture*
*How Teeth Grow*
*First Aid—Control of Breathing*
*The Blood*
*The Feet*
*Cleanliness: Bathing*
*First Aid: Carrying the Injured*
*First Aid: Life Saving and Resuscitation*
*The Living Cell*
*Muscles*
*Sewage Disposal*
*Tuberculosis*
*Home Nursing: the Bed-Bath*
*Breathing*
*Home Nursing: Special Procedures*
*Cleanliness: Keeping the Hair Clean*
*Cleanliness: Clean Hands and Face*
*The Body Framework*
*White Rats and Food*
*Good Foods: Bread*
*Good Foods: Fruits and Vegetables*
*School Children of Many Lands*

Not all of these films were made for the Society for Visual Education, because after a few years the society's then-existing films were sold to Eastman Kodak Company, for whom some of the above pictures were made. The Eastman Film Library was sold later to the *Encyclopedia Brittanica.*

It was great fun making these films. A teacher guide was printed for each film, describing the scenes and giving facts which the teacher would like to have at hand. A film strip was also made for each film with selected frames from the movie to be used in still-picture projection. A motion-picture machine was available with a gold screen which dropped down between the lamp and the film when the film was stopped to keep it from burning during a few minutes of explanation and discussion.

Early teaching films have now been largely replaced by sound films in which the voice aids in the teaching. The value of these silent films depended in large measure upon the preparation of the teacher for the film lesson. We used them constantly in the Malden studies in health education and in the teaching of school health-education methods.

I remember two evenings of film showing of special interest. One was the showing of films at an alumni dinner of M.I.T. graduates. The other was a showing of films particularly for the children who had taken part as actors and who came to Tech that evening with their parents. In announcing the films at the beginning of the program, I told the audience that, after the pictures were shown, they would have a chance to see the stars—meaning of course the children who had taken part in making the films. The delightful and naïve modesty of children was reflected by one of the boys, who came to me to ask, "When are we going outdoors to look at the stars?"

# 16

# THE GREAT UNDERWEIGHT ILLUSION

You may be interested historically (or you may not) in the nature of the once widespread program for "underweight" children and what happened to it.

In thousands of schools all over the country in the early Twenties, children were weighed and measured and their weight compared to the average weight of boys or girls of their age, and the average height as set forth in height-weight-age tables. The tables had been made by different men by taking the average weight for boys and separate average weights for girls at each age and at different heights to the nearest inch. Boys or girls whose weight was 10% or more below the weight suggested for sex, age and height in the tables were called "underweight" and given special attention to "bring them out of the underweight group."

The fallacious practice of bringing these so-called underweight children out of the underweight group might have been avoided if the tables had been given some such title as "Average weights for boys or for girls of various ages and heights." Instead, the weights given in the tables were called "normal" weights for the different ages and heights, and "10% underweight" was meant to imply a degree of emaciation or malnutrition which needed attention.

During the Twenties we were conducting a very successful experimental program in health education in the public schools of Malden ("Malden Studies in Health Education and Growth," C. E. Turner, Dr.P.H., *American Journal of Public Health,* Vol. XVIII, No. 10, Oct. 1928). The children were weighed each month because the desire to grow is a primary incentive for healthful living and because an opportunity to watch one's growth stimulated each child in maintaining good habits of food, sleep and daily hygiene. We observed many cases of excellent growth on the part of thin children; but they did not greatly change their relation to the appropriate figure in the height-age-weight table, which was then, as we said, mistakenly called "normal weight." In general, excellent growth left the thin children still thin and the stocky children still stocky. To use an analogy from the world of household pets, the greyhounds were still greyhounds and the St. Bernards still St. Bernards.

Obviously we were dealing with differences in skeletal or body build, and not with a standard structural build from which children were underweight only when they were emaciated. An interesting illustration of this fact was observed in a visit to Hawaii in the late Twenties. The schools there sought out the "underweight" children, but instead of using 10% as the break-off point for all children they put Japanese children in the underweight group if they were 8% below the "normal weight"—but the only Chinese children called underweight were those who were 12% or more below "normal weight." Chinese children were more slender and had less sturdy skeletons than Japanese children. To use 10% would show tremendous numbers of underweight Chinese children and hardly any underweight Japanese children, the school authorities said.

In studying the soundness and fallacies of this practice ("Precision and Reliability of Underweight Measurement," C. E. Turner, Dr.P.H., *American Journal of Public Health,* Vol. XIX, No. 9, Sept. 1929), several facts appeared. The suggested weights proposed in the different weight-height-age tables differed rather sharply. The "percent underweight" for the individual child jumped around because of using whole pounds, whole years of age and whole inches of height. In studying medical diagnoses of nutrition it was found that many children with a medical diagnosis of malnutrition were not 10% underweight and many of the 10%

underweight children were judged medically to be in good nutritional health.

An interesting incident caused us to check the importance of the ways in which the underweight computation was made. Another city near Boston published a school report saying that the number of children in the underweight group had been cut in half by means of the excellent school health program. I knew the Assistant Superintendent of Schools, and asked her to tell me whether any changes had been made in the method of computation. She said yes. In the beginning they used the Wood tables, but they changed to the supposedly superior Baldwin-Wood tables. They had at first used age to the nearest birthday, but they found it simpler to use the October age right through the year. They had initially weighed children with shoes on because they feared embarrassment. As the weighing program went on they weighed the children without shoes.

In order to see what these changes did to the percentage of children in the underweight group, we made these changes in the computation of underweight for 239 boys and 236 girls for whom we had complete 1922 data. Making the computation in March with the Baldwin-Wood tables and the October age without shoes, we had less than half as many children in the underweight group as when the computations were made with the Wood tables, March age to the nearest birthday, and with shoes. Any school would make a striking change in the number of underweight children if it weighed children in the fall with shoes and in March without shoes.

Obviously the *method* of computing underweight was very important in determining the size of the underweight group, and the quality of the health program was not. We found that school systems which used the underweight plan had some very unhappy, slender school children who tried hard but unsuccessfully to get out of the underweight group. One pediatrician went to different communities to conduct nutrition clinics for underweight children, but he found he could not guarantee to bring children out of the underweight group.

We wrote to Professor Baldwin, and he was so kind as to send us data on the individual children used in making the tables. Some of these "healthy children" deviated from the average by as much as 10%. This meant that, if some of the "healthy children" used in making a table could have taken a copy of the table back to school with them the day they were measured, they would have been found to be in the underweight group.

Following the presentation of the data showing that underweight was a matter of body-build and not nutrition to Professor Baldwin and Professor Wood, they withdrew the height-weight-age tables and urged the discontinuation of "underweight" programs. The director of school health in one state wrote me in some distress that we were destroying their whole state program, which was based on underweight.

We did find from our studies which weighed children every month ("Intermittency in Growth as an Index of Health Status," C. E. Turner, Dr.P.H., Ellen Lytle and Charlotte Winnemore, M.D., *American Journal of Public Health,* Vol. XXII, No. 5, May 1932) that regular and consistent growth or cessation of growth for an appreciable period was related to health status. About 10% of the elementary school children failed to gain for 3 months in succession, and as a group they had more unhygienic habits, more physical defects, and more illness than children who had gained regularly. The number of children defective in two or all three of these respects was four times as great.

# 17

## TEST-ROOM STUDIES IN WORKER EFFICIENCY

It was a mild late September morning. I was in my office by the dome in the central building at M.I.T. There was nothing to suggest the beginning of an exciting and significant adventure when the phone rang and a voice said:

"Professor Turner?"

"Yes."

"This is the President's Secretary. President Stratton wishes to speak with you on the phone. I will put him on."

"Good morning, Professor Turner. One of our graduates, Mr. Pennock, Assistant Works Manager at Western Electric in Chicago, is in my office. They have some studies under way in working efficiency. He would like advice. I told him that you teach our course in Industrial Hygiene and suggested that he come up to see you."

Mr. Pennock explained that they had carried on a study in cooperation with the illumination industry on the value of factory lighting. It had had unexpected results.

A large group of workers on a bench-type coil-winding job were separated into two smaller groups of equal size and output and placed in workrooms which were exactly alike, each with illumination of eleven-foot candles at the workbench. In one room this level was maintained while in the other the lighting was gradually reduced over a six-month period. It was thought that the reduction in output in the poorly-lighted room would be a good measure of the contribution of good lighting to the output of the worker. The lighting in the experimental room was reduced to the point at which one could hardly read a newspaper, but the output there kept ahead of that in the well-lighted room. This experiment had not been published, but it had stimulated the company to set up a test room to study the factors which really do influence output.

Mr. Pennock agreed that sharp vision was not needed on the coil-winding job and that probably the same results would not have been obtained in a needle-threading operation. I suggested, however, that the study of human behavior cannot be conducted like an experiment in physics where one factor is varied while all the others are held constant.

To illustrate this I told him of a luncheon study in high schools which had just come to my attention. Three groups of students were selected, each in a different junior high school; each group was of the same size and made up of "paired" or similar children with respect to sex, size and weight. One group had milk for the mid-morning lunch. Another had orange juice and the third group had no lunch. The experiment was to determine whether milk or orange juice contributed more to growth. The children learned of the study and all became interested in growing as fast as possible. Those who had no mid-morning lunch grew most, those who had orange juice grew next best, and those who had milk grew least.

Mr. Pennock agreed that the test room must be a biological experiment where all possible factors would be watched constantly and where changes in working conditions could be made. It was agreed that I would serve as the consultant for the test-room study and come to Chicago for three or four days each month to plan schedules and assess developments. The fee was $50 a day for time spent. This is much less than the daily income of a consultant today, but in the uninflated dollar of the Twenties it was an inviting amount. My visits were made by overnight train rides.

Mr. Pennock said they also had an interviewing program under way to learn how employees felt toward working conditions, and that he was going to the Harvard Business School to see if Dr. Elton Mayo would act as consultant to that activity. Such consulting was arranged, and I occasionally saw Dr. Mayo at Hawthorne. However, I did not participate in the interviewing program, nor did he have anything to do with the test-room activities.

In setting up the experiment, six experienced female operators, chosen at random, were removed to a small test room from the department in which they were working. Their work was the assembly of telephone relays and involved putting together a coil, an armature, contact springs, and insulators in a fixture, and securing the parts in position by means of four machine screws. They were expressly cautioned to work at a comfortable pace.

There was a hole in the bench at the right of each girl's position into which completed relays were dropped. The relay fell through a chute actuating a flapper gate. The opening of the gate closed an electrical circuit which controlled a perforating device which in turn recorded the completion of the relay by punching a hole in a moving tape. This tape moved at a rate of 1/4" per minute. The punched tape furnished a complete output record for each girl for each hour of the day.

There was no group chief in the test room, but instead a "friendly observer" of the experiment. The girls were allowed to talk and to leave the bench whenever they liked. From the output records above mentioned, we determined for each operator (1) the daily output; (2) the average hourly output for different times of day, for different days of the week and for different periods of the study; (3) average weekly output; (4) the number of defective relays; (5) the amount of repair work done.

Data concerning changes in the health, the habits, or the attitudes of the operators were secured from (1) physical examinations, (2) the comments of operators, (3) attendance irregularities, (4) occasional checks for blood-pressure and pulse-rate records, (5) vascular skin-reaction readings, (6) records of the hours of sleep, (7) social case records, (8) intelligence and dexterity tests, (9) questionnaires to reflect attitudes toward working conditions, (10) diet records over certain periods.

For details you would need to refer to a summary of these studies ("Test-Room Studies in Employee Effectiveness," C. E. Turner, *American Journal of Public Health,* June 1933), or to a more lengthy accumulation of the data. We may mention here some of the conclusions.

We came to realize that neuro-muscular fatigue is not of great importance in light industrial processes, but that the mental attitudes of the employees are of tremendous importance. The phenomenal increase in the output of the original test-room operators of from 40 per cent to 62 per cent, with less conscious expenditure of energy, indicates that a great deal more can be done to increase human productivity, with the lessening of the human energy cost (both physical and mental), without any change whatsoever in the set-up of the work itself. We know from the physical examinations of the test-room operators that their health status was not impaired. We know, from our test-room experience with these operators, that their mental tone and zest for work increased tremendously. It should be remembered that these girls were working on a piecework basis without critical supervision under the biologically-natural situation of being allowed to work at their own pace without criticism because of fluctuating output. They were not expected to meet a given output every day.

A daily 15-minute rest period did not reduce daily output. Shortening the work week did not show an increase in hourly output, but shortening the working day did show such an increase. This study has contributed to the use of the test-room method in studying working efficiency.

Apart from the statistical data from the group, we saw individual relationships of interest. For example, the output of one of the girls showed a sudden drop. It stayed down for about two weeks and then suddenly went back up to normal. Referring to the diary-type records kept by the "friendly observer" who had replaced the group chief, we found that the girl had been at odds with her mother over the period in question. She had met a new boy whom she liked but her mother objected to his different religion and would not let him come to the house. But finally the mother decided that "Gus seemed to be a good fellow" and approved the friendship. That was when her daughter's output returned to normal.

# 18

## EN ROUTE

You grandchildren have all seen at our house the globe upon which the first of three world tours was traced in a heavy black line. You may be interested in some of the odd or especially interesting things which happened in the way of tourism.

The trip in 1935 and 1936 was before organized world air travel. Our trip by boats and trains took a full calendar year of time. During the first two months I conducted a health-education study tour to Poland, Russia, Finland, Sweden and England. Naomi joined me at Le Havre the first of September, and the remaining ten months were en route.

The trip was made in large part in behalf of the World Federation of Education Associations. We had letters of introduction to their national groups, letters to M.I.T. local alumni associations, and a most useful letter to all Kodak stores around the world from President Lovejoy of Eastman Kodak, an M.I.T. graduate.

The first really unusual city was Istanbul, with its mosques, distinctive architecture, and markets—especially the jewelry market, because of the large amount of jewelry coming to Istanbul from the U.S.S.R. in the years following the Russian Revolution. Shopping was most interesting. The various pieces of jewelry were not on display as in our jewelry stores. The dealer sat behind the table in his stall. We told him what kind of jewelry we desired to see, and he had specimens brought from a back room. We were so interested in buying a star ruby that we almost missed the ferry taking us across the strait to the station from which the train to Ankara departed. The baggage had been put aboard, and I jumped on the ferry just as it was pulling away from the wharf.

Ankara was then relatively new and especially interesting as a modern city growing out of the desert. Our train from Ankara to Port Said traveled, of course, across Turkey, Syria and Israel. In Jerusalem we had the rare pleasure of having our meals in the hotel at the table with Henrietta Szold, the remarkable American Jewess who founded Hadassah in 1912.

At one place in the desert there was a unique view of a racing camel. Other passengers in our railway car told us that the camel which raced our train for a quarter of a mile was ridden by an officer of the desert police. It was a beautiful animal, and we had had no idea of the speed which this seemingly clumsy animal could develop.

At Port Said a customs officer went through our baggage and took an electric flatiron, which we thought he perhaps intended to keep. But some days later upon our return from Cairo and the Pyramids to take the boat to Bombay, he gave back our precious iron.

Upon the advice of my friend Victor Heiser, we took a P & O boat (Peninsula & Oriental) from Port Said to Bombay. Victor had said, "I think you'll like it. Of course, it is very English." We thought he meant that the crew was English, which seemed all to the good. The crew *was* English, but the line served primarily the civil service personnel traveling between India and England.

We were quite unprepared for British formality. In the dining salon we sat at large tables, and on deck we used the deck chairs; but, having no one to introduce us, we made no acquaintances and held no conversations with our fellow passengers. An odd related and subsequent incident took place in Singapore. As a professional courtesy we were invited to the home of the health officer, Dr. Scharff, for dinner, and were a bit startled to find that his wife was one of the people who had eaten at the table with us for a week or more on the boat, but whom we had never met.

India was in those days quite different from the Western World. At the World Federation of Education Association meetings in Oxford a few weeks earlier I had asked Ishbel MacDonald, the daughter of Prime Minister Sir Ramsay MacDonald, and Chairman of one of the WFEA Sections, whether I should seek a letter of introduction from the Education Department in England to educational administrators in India. She said, "No, the feeling between India and England is such that you will do well to go just as an American educator. You will be cordially received."

I spent a very pleasant afternoon with the Assistant Superintendent of Schools in Bombay, whose superior, the Superintendent, was an Englishman. During the conversation I asked whether he was interested in that post for himself. He said, "No, if I moved up to that post I would be in a predicament. Either I would have to appoint all of my relatives to jobs and spoil the school system, or I would make professional appointments and lose standing in my family."

One of my most helpful bits of advice came to me in connection with India. In London an American lady, who had read some of my writing introduced me to a Buddhist priest who had established a congregation in London. I spent two evenings with him discussing Indian customs. The second evening I asked him whether he had any advice for me personally. He said, "If I criticize you, you will be offended."

Upon being assured that I would not, he said, "Like many Americans you lack calmness. You move too rapidly in presenting your ideas. In India we feel that a person who is not calm is a young soul who is not very mature. If you wish to be highly regarded in India, you must acquire a calm demeanor and a calm presentation."

A friend in Bombay was helpful in the matter of travel. We told him that we had been advised to hire a bearer to go with us. He said, "Oh, there is no need of that. You secure bedding for your cabin on the train. You will find porters everywhere. Actually the bearer-guide kind of person may write ahead to the storekeepers he is to take you to, saying that he is coming with a golden bird." We followed his advice and found ourselves most cordially treated everywhere.

I will not weary you with details of the trip to Delhi, where we visited the palace of the Governor General; to Agra, where we were particularly fortunate to see the Taj Mahal in bright moonlight when the semi-precious stones of the building glowed most beautifully; to Allahabad and its agricultural college; and to Benares.

Our principal host in Calcutta was Sir Hassan Surrawaddy. He was a charming and remarkable man who had been Chancellor of the University of Calcutta and who was, at the time of our visit, the physician in charge of the health of the workers on the national railroad. In fact he took us out to the village where the railroad repair shops were located. Workers' houses were small, one-room or two-room structures. Sir Hassan asked if I would like to visit one and secured the permission from a man for us to go into his house. Inside there was very little furniture.

When we came out, Sir Hassan said, "You saw the woman on the bed, didn't you?"

I said, "No, I saw a big pile of rugs on the bed but no woman."

He said, "There was a woman rolled up inside the rugs. She is pregnant and is purposely perspiring as a traditional, supposedly hygienic measure in pregnancy. Actually this is, of course, very bad for her because she will be weak and debilitated when the time for childbirth arrives and she will find delivery very difficult."

Sir Hassan invited us to dinner and promised to visit us on his forthcoming trip to America. He did later come to our house, having sent us a message from the boat regarding the time of arrival. Two differences between American and Indian customs appeared on that visit.

The first difference had to do with bathing customs. The Indian uses a small room with a tiled floor, a tank of clear water, and a dipper. He pours water over himself, soaps and rinses himself. The water is carried off in a drain from the tile floor.

Sir Hassan arrived at our house in midafternoon, and while I went away in the car to get other dinner guests, he took the opportunity for a bath. Our bathroom had a tiled floor and a tub. Doubtless Sir Hassan thought it would certainly be all right to bathe Indian fashion on the tiled bathroom floor of a public health person. Mrs. Turner was downstairs arranging for dinner when water began to drip from the ceiling beneath the bathroom. There was nothing she could do but wait in the downstairs hall until she heard Sir Hassan return to his room, whereupon she rushed to the bathroom with an armful of towels to stop the drip.

The other difference related to the European and Asiatic habit of leaving shoes outside the bedroom door to be cleaned and polished by the houseboy. We had no houseboy, of course, but when Mrs. Turner came upstairs, as the last member of the household to retire, she saw Sir Hassan's shoes outside the door. Feeling that we must not be behind India in our hospitality, she took the shoes and polished them, and put them back at the door.

The only remark concerning this development came when I was taking Sir Hassan back to the train. He said, "Oh, Professor, I forgot to leave any money for the servants."

Our staff being comprised of one maid, I said, "That was not necessary. Actually, we don't do that much in this country."

Whereupon he gave me a fifty-cent piece and said, "Well, at least let me give you this for the poor devil who shined my shoes." I did not tell him that the "poor devil" was my wife.

One of the striking adventures in this tour was a train trip from Calcutta to Darjeeling in the Himalayas. We visited among other places a very simple mountain temple. A horn, some eight feet long, was suspended, pointing out over the valley. The Lama had a container in the shape of an old-fashioned hot-water tank which an assistant priest turned slowly by an attached crank. The bottom of the tank rested on an iron spike which in turn rested upon a seashell. We were told that the tank was filled with written prayers, and that so long as they were moving, they would constantly receive the attention of the Almighty.

An oddity in the hotel at Penang was the headwaiter who identified himself by wearing a large button about the size of the center of a sunflower, saying "No. 1 Boy."

The trip from Penang to Bangkok was on the Royal Siamese Express, a very comfortable train with European-style passenger cabins. We expected some courtesies from the government because the father and mother of the king had both been my students; but we did not expect these courtesies to start so soon. A few miles out of Penang a young man in the military uniform of a captain came to our cabin. "Are you Professor Turner?" said he. "The government is expecting you. I shall be in the cabin ahead. Please let me know if there is anything you wish."

One of the most interesting nights we ever spent on shipboard was enroute between Bangkok and Singapore. The boat we were on carried freight as well as passengers. There was a delay in getting the boat loaded and in leaving Bangkok. The result was that we arrived near the mouth of the Menam River at low tide and there was not enough water to carry us over the bar. The boat stopped for the night at a place called Mosquito Point. We saw the crew eating early, and when we went to dinner by lamplight, we knew why. Insects were attracted by the light, and it was next to impossible to get a bit of food from the plate to the mouth without having insects attached. Through the night we heard noises from the jungle animals, especially the chattering of monkeys and the indistinct cries of other animals.

Our longest boat trip was from Soerabaja to Manila on a freight boat where we were two of the eight or ten passengers. We ate at the table with the captain and the ship's doctor. The second day out we heard a noise which seemed familiar to me from my boyhood, and I said to the doctor, "This sounds like someone is killing a pig."

"You're right, someone *is* killing a pig," said the doctor. "We have a few hundred Chinese men on the lower deck. In Chinese culture it is highly desirable for a man to go back to his native country to die. Workmen have little money, and I will show you tomorrow how we can carry them at little expense."

The next day the doctor took us below deck where we saw a great area fenced off with heavy iron grill fencing like that used in the construction of prisons. One of the foods supplied there was a kind of stew produced by killing a pig daily, cutting up the pork, and cooking it in a stew.

Interest was added on this trip by the stop of a few hours at the Celibes and at Borneo. As we pulled into the harbor at Manila, we saw some twenty people waiting on the dock and wondered what it was all about, until, as we got nearer, we found the group to be made up of former Philippine students at M.I.T. and their friends.

One of the world's most delightful boat trips was on the *Asama Maru* from Japan to Hawaii. The perfect service, the delicious food, the days on the deck in the sun, are never to be forgotten.

## 19

## JAVA AND BALI

On the afternoon of January 3, 1936, we ended our ten-day visit to Singapore and took the Dutch boat *Ophir* for Batavia. We crossed the Equator early in the morning of January 4 and arrived in Batavia on January 5, beginning a stay of 16 days, crossing Java from west to east and enjoying a side trip to Bali.

Language on the boat was Dutch and Malay, but many stewards spoke some English. There was no trouble with language, but we did run into a problem in the use of clothing. At breakfast the first day out I wore white duck trousers and a white Russian blouse. A half-hour after breakfast, a steward rapped at our cabin door and said, "The Captain's compliments, sir, but he requests you not to wear pajamas at breakfast."

I assured him with great dignity that I had not done so, saying, "Has the Captain never been in Russia?"

He bowed and retired, returning twenty minutes later to say, "The Captain's apologies, sir. He has never been in Russia."

Dr. John Lee Hydrick, who had made a visit of several days at M.I.T. and the Malden health education program a few years earlier, met us at the boat. He was carrying on a rural health and health education project in Java and took us across the island, showing us beautiful scenery, museums, temples and health programs. The most unique and interesting of our experiences were in studying village life and the public health work which Dr. Hydrick was doing. His project has been beautifully described in his book entitled *Inten-*

*sive Rural Hygiene Work in Netherlands, India.*

The first day's drive had an interesting incidental experience. Dr. Hydrick stopped the car to pick up a melon from a roadside fruit seller. The melon, which looked innocent enough, was a *durian*—a fruit which is most unusual in odor and taste, being stronger than the strongest overripe cheese you can imagine. Dr. Hydrick told us to put a very small piece in the mouth, but even so it seemed that we would never get rid of that taste. Dr. Hydrick had brought some Dentyne gum to help. Hotels have signs prohibiting bringing durians into the rooms. And yet we found that people become extremely fond of this melon and get together for durian parties.

The principal health worker being trained by Dr. Hydrick for use in the village was the *mantri.* The word means a technically-trained person. Most of the mantris were men; a few were women. Their health-education activities with the villagers had resulted in the building of latrines, in making costless toothbrushes and nail brushes of coconut bark, in making covers of bamboo to protect food from flies, in teaching the boiling of drinking water, the washing of hands before eating, etc.

We accompanied a mantri on a house visit. The houses are made of bamboo and are suitable for the climate of Java, which lies only five to eight degrees south of the Equator. The mantri sat on a flat bench with members of the family. Java has traditionally had a caste system, and they would be embarrassed if the mantri stood or sat on a chair while they squatted on a bench or the floor. He spoke high Javanese to the adult members of the family and low Javanese to the children.

He told us that he was accompanied by a member of the village government on his first visit. This assured the family that he had permission to work in the village and that he could be trusted. In his educational activities he used models, photographs and charts which he put into the hands of the family while he developed an informal discussion.

A most patient discussion-leader, he told us that the majority of the adults were illiterate and that repeated visits were needed in the promotion of any particular activity. At the schools the children made long bamboo water containers with many outlets as a source of water for hand-washing.

On Saturday mornings Dr. Hydrick had staff meetings with role-playing as a means of increasing the skill of the workers. We saw a Saturday-morning session of the mantris. One of the young men took the part of a mantri and other young men and young women took the parts of members of the family. The mantri presented his house-visit educational material. The members of the family asked questions and participated in the discussion. They presented problems which the visiting mantri must solve.

Another activity was the training of village women to become *doekoens* and deliver babies. These educational activities were carried out by qualified midwives. The doekoens were taught to wash their hands properly, clean their nails, to care for the cord properly, to boil instruments, to wash the baby properly. They were taught to call the midwife or the doctor if the birth seemed abnormal.

Gradually the people have been taught the value of the midwife, so that skilled services have continually increased. We saw a teaching demonstration in which one of the doekoens took the part of a midwife. The "mother" lay down on the dirt floor in accord with the old customs and the belief that the baby would gain strength from the earth. First the "midwife" persuaded the mother to get off the floor and lie on a clean bench. A doll was used to take the place of the baby. The midwife washed her hands thoroughly, and boiled some water to use in washing the "baby." She removed the baby from under the skirt of the expectant mother, cut the "cord," and carried out the other birth activities, including washing both the baby and the mother.

There were interesting stories about the Sultan of Solo who controlled territory in the center of the island. His servants had had the habit of washing rice in a highly polluted canal before cooking it. They were told that they should wash the rice in boiled water. They did so and, having done as they were told, they took it down to the polluted canal and washed it as usual.

We did not visit the Sultan's palace but saw an automobile filled with his wives in Soerabaja. At least we were told that they were the Sultan's wives coming in to shop.

The zoo at Soerabaja was of special interest. The six-foot Commodo lizard was a startling sight. We were taking colored movies and following the picture of a beautiful peacock. We took one of an albino peacock. When we showed these pictures we always had a demonstration of what a beautiful color is white. People enjoyed the color of peacock No. 1, but the audience always gasped when the all-white peacock appeared on the screen.

A few days in Bali was a side trip. We landed at the north side of the island, which was already Europeanized, and took a bus across the island to Denpasar on the south shore. The raising of rice in the little valleys and on the terraced hillsides contributed remarkable landscapes in which the water reflected the blue of the sky, colored with the green blades of rice extending an inch or so above the water.

In 1936 Southern Bali was little changed from its ancient customs. Dress for girls and women was limited to an apron or skirt. Dress for men was limited to a jockstrap in most cases. Women did most of the work and cockfighting was a major activity for men. Woodcarving and the making of fine handwrought jewelry was well developed.

One of the most delightful activities was the dancing of youth in traditional form, telling the story of a princess who was stolen by an evil spirit and rescued by a hero. The dancers appeared to be about eleven or twelve years old and wore elaborate costumes. They danced inside a rectangular line made by older boys and girls seated on the ground, also in formal costumes. It seemed like a reversal of Western customs in that these girls *put on* clothes for the dance. The music for the dance was furnished by a *gamelan* (xylophone-type) orchestra, the musicians sitting on the ground.

We had two days in Soerabaja after our return to Java before embarking on the boat to Manila. It was made especially memorable by an invitation to rice *tafel.* When we were all comfortably seated at the restaurant tables, the parade of twenty-one neatly attired waiters began their march, each bringing us a different fruit, soup, fish, meat, rice or dessert. There was so much delicious food as to be temporarily incapacitating, but it was a fitting end to a fascinating visit to the island.

## 20

## PRE-REVOLUTIONARY CHINA OF THE 1930's

We were fortunate to spend a month in China during our World Tour in 1935-36—prior to the war between China and Japan and the revolution in China. Let me write down for you not a diary of the trip but stories of some of its more interesting happenings.

We came to China from the Philippines early in February. The stewards on the boat from Manila to Hong Kong were Japanese, and one of the officers was good enough to tell us that we must not give a gratuity to the steward in the form of "raw" money. We must put our bills in a sealed envelope.

In Shanghai, Mrs. Turner stayed for two weeks while my friend and former student, Dr. C. K. Chu, and I went on a big circle tour set up by the Minister of Health, Dr. J. Heng Liu. We spent a few days in Nanking arranging for visits to the various provincial health officers, and then went to Peking, Hanchow, Chungking, Changsha, Nanchang, Foochow, Hangchow, and back to Shanghai. Mrs. Turner joined us and we returned to Nanking and Peking for a week or so before going north through Manchuria to Korea.

Let me first tell the story of the wolf-belly fur coat which all of you grandchildren have seen. Nanking seemed very cold to me, coming as we had from the Tropics. So Dr. Chu and I went to the furrier to buy a coat. We were visiting elementary schools in which there was no heat, and in which each child wore three or four coats. The furrier had a tremendous variety of furs waiting to be made up. An American-type coat appealed to me—such as were worn in those days to football games. Dr. Chu did not tell me that in

China only women wore coats with fur on the outside. Men's coats were always made with fur on the inside. Most intriguing was a gray fur which the merchant said was Siberian wolf-bellies. In a couple of days he had made me an excellent coat of this material. It had no pockets on the outside, which men's coats probably would have had, but in every other respect it was quite satisfactory.

An amusing element was that the picture I presented when wearing the coat—that of a foreign devil in a woman's coat—led to great hilarity among the Chinese people who saw me. On part of our trip to the interior we were joined by Dr. Y. Y. Lung, a provincial health officer and a former student. He had a great sense of humor, and one of his delights at an occasional station-stop of the train was to put on my "woman's coat" and run up and down the platform, to the great delight of all of the travelers present.

Our purchases were all interesting. I remember the introduction to bargaining from the wife of an M.I.T. graduate who had invited us to his house for tea. I asked her, "Should I start by offering half the price he asks?" and she said, "Oh, no, start by offering one-tenth."

Our most extensive purchase was in Chinese rugs, of which we bought some fifteen or twenty. I remember so well the day of selecting rugs at the Fette Rug Company. Mr. Fette was a young man who went to China to teach, following the completion of his education in the United States. His wife sent individual Chinese rugs to some of her friends. Out of this she developed an export rug business which was so much more lucrative than teaching school that her husband joined her. In their showrooms were piles of rugs more than four feet high, and two Chinese boys turned them back one after another while we made our selections. Their purchase was 35 years ago as I write this, and they still look like new. Chinese rugs are rare at this time, and their value is several times their purchase price.

An experience of special interest was our visit to the Medical College at Changsha, which has been known here in

America as "Yale in China." The dean was a delightful physician who had studied medicine in Japan and married there. He and his wife had us for dinner. In the evening I gave a lecture on health education to senior medical-school students. There was no heat in the lecture room and the lecture was given in my wolf-belly fur coat, through a very capable interpreter. When the dean, Dr. Chu, and I later finished our discussions on public health, it was nearly midnight, but the dean's wife was ready to bring us a cup of tea to put a gracious end to the evening.

You grandchildren have slept under one or more of the five silk and silk-embroidered bedspreads and seen the various silk-embroidered pillow covers which came from Changsha. The wife of the dean took me shopping the second morning of our visit to select needlework from a perfectly marvelous assortment. It seems that Changsha was the center of this sort of thing.

In those days each province had one or more things for which it was famous. On the evening of an overnight train trip Dr. Chu said to me, "About midnight the train will stop at a city where I have relatives. This province is famous for smoked ham. My cousin will come on the train and put a smoked ham under your berth. I hope it will not disturb you."

Were you ever in the midst of people in an exciting situation but unable to communicate with anyone? I was in that situation once in the midst of rickshaws. Dr. Chu and I got off the train and took our baggage to the edge of the platform where there were some twenty-five or thirty rickshaws, each with its runner. Dr. Chu put our baggage in one rickshaw and sent off the boy to our hotel. He climbed into another rickshaw, put me in a third, and took off down the street, around the corner, and out of sight. Immediately a fight broke out as to whose passenger I would be. There was some physical violence and an unlimited amount of verbiage. The bad part of my situation was that I did not know a word of Chinese and no one around me knew a word of English.

There was nothing I could do except to sit still and hope that Dr. Chu would come back for me. He was back in ten or twelve minutes, having found that my rickshaw was not following him, and the "tempest in a teapot" was over.

One of the most delightful aspects of China was the food. In Nanking Dr. Chu took me to two or three delicious dinners with other doctors. At the first dinner we were served deliciously mild Chinese wine. At the second dinner there was a change arranged by Dr. Chu's sense of humor. The wine tasted mild and smooth, but it was obviously different in authority. I suddenly realized that I must either stop drinking or stop talking.

The really unsurpassed food anywhere in the world is Peking duck. Naomi and I were invited to such a dinner as members of a dinner party of some half a dozen people. First we assembled in a pleasant waiting room where the restaurant manager brought us three very fat ducks for our choice. They were all perfect birds, but we selected one as a matter of formality. We were left to chat for a few minutes when a boy brought us each a serving of soup made from the brain of the duck.

We were told about how these ducks were fattened. They were kept in small pens to limit their exercise; and, in order to increase their caloric intake, rice was pushed down their throats after they had finished their normal meal. They were so fat that when they were roasted between a fire and a brick wall, they basted themselves. The skin was brown and crisp. In serving the duck each piece of meat had some of the skin attached and was eaten with a rich and delicious dressing.

But we were talking about purchases. Others were in art, including a modest amount of jade and a few pieces of ivory, including especially Quanyin, the Goddess of Mercy, which you have seen at our house. She is about a foot tall and is made from the end of an elephant tusk. These tusks, you know, are two of the elephant's teeth. At the bottom of the statue one can see the end of the dental cavity. We were a little surprised to find that the cost of having a wooden niche made for the statue in America was more than the cost of the statue in China.

The social contacts in China were thoroughly delightful. They included a visit to the classical Chinese theater. There were many visits with former students. Miss Chow (Chow Mei Yu), a nurse who had studied health education at Tech and who later as the Director of Nurses in the Chinese Army became the world's first woman general, spent several hours with us, as did Thomas Yuan, a former student in the United States who was Director of Physical Education at Peking University. Several other former students in public health in the United States met with us in discussion groups, and our last week in China was given over to a national health-education conference.

This conference was established by the Minister of Health, Dr. J. Heng Liu, and organized by Dr. Chu, who was then serving as the National Director of Health and Medical Education. The conference involved a considerable group since most of the provinces were represented as well as the National Ministry of Health. It was the first health-education conference China had had, and because the Japanese war and the revolution soon intervened, it was up to this time the only such conference. Plans were made for constructive national and local developments in health education.

One of our happiest surprises was with the American Customs Service. We stopped off a week in Hawaii, which meant that we went through customs in Honolulu rather than in San Francisco. We had carefully listed the prices paid for each of our purchases, but we found that there was no customs due on the majority of them because they were over one hundred years old.

The following are quotes from letters to Mrs. Turner in Shanghai while Dr. Chu and I were making the journey to the interior of the country:

> *Peking, Sunday evening.* Shall have very busy schedule. Must give one lecture at Central Normal University.

Some teas, dinners, etc. Visits to schools and other universities.

*Hangkow, Friday, March 20.* I am glad that you did not try to come on this trip. I have suffered more hours with the cold since I left Shanghai than in any ordinary winter at home. You see, most meals are eaten Chinese style, which means in an unheated room with coats on. But the Chinese wear heavy underwear and sheepskin coats which reach to the ground. Bring them into a heated house and they perspire like rain. The next time I go to a cold and developing country, I shall first ask how men's clothes are made, and when, if ever, they take off any of these heavy garments. The fur coat helped me some but a man in a light suit and BVD's under conditions when everyone around him is in wool and sheepskin is bound to freeze his legs off.

We could not go from Changsha to Nanchang by car because the roads are impassable. We had to stay over a day, then take the train back here last night.

Some good school medical work is being started but the educational side is not well advanced. Education in general is the 3 R's. Most schools have no heat. Frozen hands is one of the most common items for treatment in school clinics. There are two, three, or four-coat days.

Lectured in Hangkow Tuesday evening. Thursday evening I lectured at Yale-in-China Medical School in Changsha (in fur coat, no hat). Wind blew through the room straight from Siberia. Very nice people in Changsha.

Dr. Lung and Dr. Wang are with us now, having decided to accompany us to Nanking in order to be there for the health education conference.

*Hangkow, Sunday evening:* Terrible dust storm Friday. Very cold. Friday and Friday night dust covered the floor like snow.

Saw Miss Chow. She will probably come to Nanking. Met Mrs. Chen who is very nice. The Chens have three beautiful children. They are working in the mass education movement.

# 21

## DR. YOSHIDA AND VISITS TO JAPAN

My first contact with Dr. Yoshida, the distinguished Director of Research in the Japanese Imperial Institute for Research in Physical Education, was in 1929. He came to Geneva, Switzerland, to present a paper before the Health Education Section of the World Federation of Education Associations. I was then serving as Section Chairman, and George Milson, Director of Junior Red Cross activities for the International Red Cross, was Secretary. The paper was written in English, but Dr. Yoshida's pronunciation was so unclear that the audience could not understand what he was saying. Some of the audience motioned to me that I should stop his presentation. Of course such a step with its consequent loss of face for a distinguished scholar who had come halfway around the world was inconceivable. Dr. Yoshida finished his paper, but he clearly understood the situation. He had the paper printed overnight and presented copies to the members of the section next day.

A lifelong friendship began at these meetings. Dr. Yoshida spent a few days at M.I.T. on his way back to Japan. I recall his comments regarding then existing contrasts. One day coming back to my office from the lunchroom he observed the great number of automobiles in the parking lot and asked, "To whom do all these automobiles belong?"

"Students," I replied.

"Students!" said Dr. Yoshida. "In Tokyo University not one full professor has his own automobile."

In 1936 he arranged a series of health-education lectures for me in Japan under the auspices of the Imperial School

Hygiene Association and the Japanese Federation of Life Insurance Companies. The former provided professional dignity and the latter provided money. Dr. Yoshida, Dr. K. Saito, Dean of the School of Public Health, and Dr. Y. Nozu, a former student of mine in health education, served as interpreters.

In advance of this series of lectures in Tokyo, Kobe, Osaka and other cities, the Japanese had translated my *Principles of Health Education,* which had been published in English in 1932. Later they translated *School Health and Health Education,* the first English edition of which appeared in 1947.

The visit to Japan in 1936 provided many hospitable, cultural and fascinating experiences for Mrs. Turner and myself. We usually lodged in typical Japanese inns, leaving our shoes outside and enjoying the *tatami,* Japanese furniture and Japanese menu. The mayor of Kobe gave us a most delightful luncheon prior to my lecture to teachers and school officials. Tea ceremonies were numerous and delightful. When we began to use chopsticks, I thought I could never get used to them. But after eating with them for a couple of months, silver knives and forks seemed positively heavy and clumsy.

One day Dr. Yoshida said to me, "Professor Turner, I wish to ask you a question. If you wish to say no, please say no. Would you like to have purification ceremony in Shinto shrine?" I was somewhat startled by being invited to accept this unusual privilege. However, our church has open communion, and it occurred to me in accepting that it would have been natural for me to invite Dr. Yoshida to participate in communion out of his respect for the Christian religion without any implication that he had changed his religious affiliation.

It was a very interesting ceremony. Dr. Yoshida and another physician accompanied me to one of the oldest Shinto shrines. A young assistant priest, wearing typical apparel of hat and cloak, met us at the outer door and escorted us to the inner room of the temple. The doctors remained at the door of this room. I proceeded to the center of the room and knelt at a small shrine. I had been given a beautiful bouquet of white roses tied in white silk ribbon as I entered the sacred edifice, and I laid these before me on the altar-like structure. The priest said prayers at the far end of the room before elaborate and beautiful altars, and then came to me in the center of the room to say additional prayers. Following this I arose and walked backward to the door from which I had entered. I have never been quite sure why Dr. Yoshida arranged this privilege; but it certainly contributed to my appreciation of Japanese culture.

At the time of Dr. Yoshida's death in the 50's, his son wrote to me of the loss of his father, saying that his father's friendship with me had meant so much that he would like to continue the relationships between the two families. This we have done. In a visit to Japan in behalf of WHO and Unesco in 1962, the Yoshida family, consisting of Dr. Yoshida's widow, his sons, his youngest son's wife and his grandchildren, invited Mrs. Turner and myself for a most cordial family dinner.

In the period 1962-64 I had intimate contact with health and education authorities in Japan in connection with the WHO-Unesco study which resulted in the Unesco publication entitled *Planning for Health Education in Schools*. The preliminary draft of this report in English was sent to Japan; and the day these copies were mailed, Mrs. Turner and I started for the trip through the Middle East and Far East to consult with leaders in school health education. We reached Japan about three weeks after leaving Paris, to find that the Japanese had already translated this 120-page document and scheduled an all-day meeting for me with the professors of health education of fifteen leading universities. I later met separately with the Minister of Health, the Minister of Education, the National Director of Physical Education, and the Dean of the School of Public Health. My last full day in Japan was given over to a meeting of some thirty or more of the leaders in health education who had prepared suggestions for the revision and improvement of the draft copy of the study. When the final report was published in 1966 (in English, French and Spanish) Japan was the first country to publish an edition in their own language.

Some of you grandchildren may have seen mementoes from Japan, including the Samurai sword, the short sword of old Japan, and the highly-decorated lacquer message box such as was used by the Shoguns a thousand years ago. When we returned from Japan, we brought *tatami* and made the former nursery into a Japanese room. I mentioned our plan to do this to the President of one of the life insurance companies at a tea we gave at the Imperial Hotel the day before leaving. We were surprised and startled, not to say embarrassed, to receive from him a few hours later a half-dozen floor cushions for our Japanese room.

# 22

## THAILAND

At the beginning of the 1920-21 school year, Professor Sedgwick called me to his office to meet Prince Songkla of Thailand and help him register as a graduate student. The prince had a long name and many titles, one of which was Duke of Songkla, one of the districts of Thailand. He preferred to be called just Mr. Songkla because, as he said, "Mr. is the highest title you have in America, and that's the way I would prefer to be addressed."

Mr. Songkla had a superior mind as a student. I saw quite a bit of him because he made a study of the public health aspects of the tuberculosis problem under my supervision.

You know of King Chulalonkorn, who was the last of the polygamous kings of Thailand. Prince Songkla was the son of Chulalonkorn by his No. 2 wife. There were two sons by the No. 1 wife, so it did not seem likely that Prince Songkla would ever become king. Actually, but for his untimely death he would have been king. But I am getting ahead of my story.

While studying at Tech, Prince Songkla met a Siamese girl of noble birth who was studying at Simmons College. He arranged for her to come to Tech for a summer course in health education. A few months after that they decided to be married. He took his chamberlain and she took her lady-in-waiting, and they returned to Siam. He decided to come back to America and study medicine. Their first two children were born here. I visited them frequently in their modest apartment, but I did not know that the baby I was seeing was a future king.

A year or two after returning to Siam, Prince Songkla

died of a kidney ailment. Soon after that the reigning king passed away and his brother withdrew from the throne because of serious eye difficulty. The succession then passed to the older son of Prince Songkla, who ruled under the guidance of three regents.

When Mrs. Turner and I were in Siam in 1935 we were entertained by the senior regent, Mr. Sukhum. Dr. Medha, who had been Director of Government Students in America, and Lady Medha accompanied us to the dinner. The residence of the Sukhum family was on the second floor, and as we reached the top stair, Lady Medha dropped to her knees. I was startled at this apparent accident but saw immediately that it was intentional. It was a gesture of respect to Regent Sukhum, who represented the king.

We sat in a waiting room for a bit and were served glasses of cold, clear water brought to us by boys who crossed the floor on their knees rather than walking. The dinner was most formal, most elaborate and most gracious.

There was another contact with Mr. Sukhum's family. While Prince Songkla was studying at M.I.T., he came to me one morning to ask whether I could render a favor to his government. He presented me with a cable saying, "It pleases his Majesty the King of Siam that Prassart Sukhum should learn to make the moving picture." The prince knew that I had been making educational films, and it was arranged that I should guide the program of Prassart in America. His sojourn in a motion picture laboratory and later with a production company was arranged. He struggled hard in improving his English and wrote to me regularly. In one letter he described his schedule and ended by saying, "I guess you will think I didn't wasted my time at all, I'll say."

Upon his return to Thailand, Prassart directed the motion picture interests of the government and also supervised a brick factory. He arranged to free his whole time for the ten days we were in his country and took us everywhere, including visits to the palaces, temples, shops, and the lapidary section of Bangkok where hundreds of zircons were being cut.

We must not leave the Thailand story without describing the trip to see the Angkor Wat, the famous assemblage of temples and shrines in Cambodia which was then a part of French Indo-China. It was an all-day journey from Bangkok to Angkor-Thom. We left at 7:30 in the morning and arrived at 8 in the evening, spending the forenoon in a train ride to the border and much of the afternoon in a small bus from the border to the village near the temple.

This was wild country. A stationmaster on the railroad had been killed by a tiger the year before. Coming back we left at 4 o'clock in the morning. Fires were burning in front of small huts in the forest; the driver told us that they were for protection against animals. The hotel where we stopped, however, was not at all primitive. It was a typically Parisian French establishment of modern structure with dining tables covered by spotless linen and with a French menu, including a long list of the best French wines.

The Wat itself is a rambling structure, said to have been built between the 9th and 13th centuries, probably by people from Java and Southern India. The stones of the buildings are not held together by mortar and the buildings themselves consist of temples, monasteries and monuments. They represent different cultures and religions, and contained over 100 carved heads of Seva and Bayon. The middle chambers have many statues of Buddha. There are Chinese-type lions. One building had four elephant statues. There are human figures holding snakes. When we were there men were clearing trees which had overgrown temple structures. Today (March 1972), as I write this, war rages about the Wat. As you read this the Wat may be either restored or destroyed.

We visited Thailand twice after 1935. One visit was in 1962 in behalf of WHO and Unesco, and the other was in 1966 as director of a world study-tour in health education.

# 23

## THE NATIONAL FOUNDATION AND THE CONQUEST OF POLIOMYELITIS

What public health experience could be more exciting than watching and participating in the conquest of a communicable disease? Such an experience was mine as Assistant to the President of the National Foundation for Infantile Paralysis from 1947 to 1958 (except for a few weeks following my retirement under the age rule and prior to an urgent request from Mr. O'Connor to come back and help out for a bit).

I had gone to the school of Public Health at the University of California at the end of World War II as the first Professor of Health Education. My appointment was as visiting professor for one to three years. At the end of one year I terminated the assignment because of my severe allergy to poison oak, in spite of a very pleasant university experience and the desire of President Sproule and Dean Brown that I should remain at California. It was then that I went to the National Foundation.

The conquest of polio was one of the great public health achievements of the century. The victory came under the leadership of one man, Basil O'Connor. All of us on the staff were deeply privileged to be members of his team.

There were several remarkable elements in the war waged by the Foundation against the disease. One was the magnitude of the problem and the program. In 1952, for example, there were 57,879 new polio cases and approximately 80,000 patients were receiving financial assistance in securing treatment of the disease. Altogether the Foundation spent approximately $280,000,000 to aid patients who needed financial assistance. In addition the foundation spent some $33,000,000 for research and $29,000,000 for the professional education of virologists, physical therapists, and other workers in the field of medicine.

It was of course the *research* which led directly to the conquest of polio. In the early 1940's the possibility of a vaccine seemed very remote for three reasons: (1) Scientists did not know how many varieties or strains of the virus were involved. (2) The only place to grow the virus was in the central nervous system of monkeys, and of course only limited quantities could be produced. (3) It was not known how the virus got into the nerve tissue. Blood samples had been taken at the first signs of paralysis but no virus had been found in the blood.

Research brought new and important knowledge. (1) An intensive worldwide investigation showed that there are three strains of the virus. Using all three strains would produce a complete vaccine.

(2) Dr. Enders found a way to grow the virus in the test tube.

(3) It was discovered that the virus *is* in the blood for a brief time before entering the nervous system. This period of viremia occurs so long before paralysis appears that it had not been discovered in earlier blood tests upon patients.

These discoveries opened the way for the production of the killed virus vaccine by Dr. Salk, and later the production of an attenuated virus vaccine by Dr. Sabin. In 1953 Dr. Salk tested his killed virus vaccine with over 400 children, including his own, in the Pittsburgh area, and an extensive evaluation of the vaccine followed in 1954.

A thrilling day was spent at the University of Michigan, April 12, 1955, when several of us from the Foundation joined national leaders in public health to hear the final report of the evaluation studies, which had involved over 1,800,000 children in 211 areas of 44 states. These studies showed clearly the effectiveness of the vaccine, and they were followed by a national vaccination program under the leadership of the Foundation and involving also the American Medical Association, public health authorities, and the public schools of the country. The number of cases reported to the Public Health Service was 38,476 in 1954, 27,985 in 1955, 15,140 in 1956, 5,894 in 1957. Today one rarely hears of a case.

The conquest of polio meant much to everyone, and especially to those of us who were in the midst of the battle, working constantly with severely crippled children, youth and adults. I remember being sent to arrange more extensive medical service for a patient about twenty years old with almost complete paralysis who could never be left alone in the hospital room because of the danger that chest and throat spasms might stop her breathing. Some of these polio patients belonged to the group of the world's bravest people. The terror of the disease was an important factor in the establishment of local chapters and March of Dimes programs in the states and local areas of the country.

My own functions with the Foundation were mainly concerned with policies and programs, and especially with relationships to schools and colleges. We maintained contact with key educators, interpreting to them the Foundation program of patient care, educational activities, and fundraising. The scope of these relationships is shown by the following list of organizations involved:

1. U.S. Office of Education
2. National Education Association, including the Central Office and also:
    a. Council of Chief State School Officers
    b. American Association of School Administrators
    c. National Association of Secondary School Principals
    d. Department of Elementary School Principals
    e. Department of Rural Education
    f. American Association for Health, Physical Education and Recreation

3. Catholic Schools
   National Catholic Education Association, including the Central Office and also:
   a. Superintendent's Department
   b. Department of Colleges and Universities
   c. Department of Secondary Schools
   d. Department of Special Education
4. Private Schools (National Council of Independent Schools)
5. Seventh Day Adventists (Department of Education)
6. United Lutheran Church (Board of Higher Education)
7. National Union of Christian Schools
8. Protestant Episcopal Church (Department of Education)
9. National School Boards Association
10. American School Health Association
11. American Student Health Association (College Physicians and Directors of Student Health)
12. National Federation of State High School Athletic Associations

In addition we maintained contact with national youth groups which were active in the campaign against the disease. These groups included: American Legion Boy's Nation, American Legion Auxiliary Girl's Nation, B'nai Brith Youth Organizations, Boy Scouts of America, Campfire Girls, 4-H Clubs, Future Farmers, Future Homemakers, Girl Scouts of America, Jack & Jill Teenagers, Junior Red Cross, National Association of Colored Girls, National Association of Student Councils, National Council of Catholic Youth, National Grange Youth, National Jewish Welfare Board (youth division), New Farmers, New Homemakers, Salvation Army (youth group), United Christian Youth, The Volunteers of America (youth group), Young Men's Christian Association and Young Women's Christian Association.

Contact with these groups at their national meetings was most stimulating. I remember especially addressing the National Council of Catholic Youth, where there were some 2,000 young people and where the other speakers were Cardinal Spellman and Richard M. Nixon, then the Vice-President.

One of the greatest privileges throughout this decade of work with the Foundation was the privilege of working directly and closely with Basil O'Connor. I cherish the following letter which he sent to me when I retired in 1955 (for a few weeks at that time, as it turned out):

January 27, 1956

Dr. Clair E. Turner
19 Village Lane
Arlington 74, Massachusetts

Dear Dr. Turner:

As you bring to a close your work with the National Foundation for Infantile Paralysis, I want to express to you my appreciation for the important contributions you have made in your ten years of association with the organization.

These have been unusually interesting years which have been marked by outstanding progress in our fight against poliomyelitis. It has been a fight on many fronts and you have been one of the effective workers in that fight. Your rich experience and many contacts with educators throughout the world as well as within this country have made easier the acceptance of our program to the point where it is well established within the schools and well accepted by education leaders. This was of particular help to us in the last few years when we found it necessary to work more closely than ever before with the schools of this country in carrying out the field trial of the Salk poliomyelitis vaccine and the subsequent poliomyelitis vaccination activities. The financial support which has come to the Foundation from schools has been in substantial measure I know a reflection of this continuing effort on your part.

But more than that, you have brought wisdom based on broad knowledge and extensive experience to the counsel you have given to me and to the members of our staff as we have worked together on program activities over the years.

I know that you are asking that your services with the National Foundation be brought to a close to enable you to devote more time to your many other interests. May I at this time, therefore, wish you continuing vigor and good health in the years ahead. Although you are now officially leaving the staff of the National Foundation, I feel confident that we shall always have in you a good friend and willing counsel.

Sincerely yours,
/s/ Basil O'Connor
President

24

# COMMUNITY ORGANIZATION FOR HEALTH EDUCATION

As health-education programs developed, broadened, and emerged from classroom programs in the schools and publicity in the adult community, it became obvious that many health education programs were demanding community action. In the health-education section of the American Public Health Association, we thought it desirable to study such programs and the community organization involved. We asked the Health Officers Section to join us in forming a joint committee on community organization for health education. As chairman of the committee I was able to secure a grant from the Charles H. Hood Educational Trust.

Our program involved two steps. First we wrote to each state health officer in the country and to each state superintendent of schools, asking them for the names of any communities in their state in which the local health department and school department had cooperated in health-education or health-promotion activities, with or without the participation of voluntary health agencies.

The second step was the actual visitation and study of selected communities by a health-education specialist. Philip L. Riley, a former student in the Department of Biology and Public Health at M.I.T., then serving as Director of Health Education for the Cleveland public schools, was engaged to make the study. He actually visited and studied 72 such programs. His investigations and report to the committee resulted in a 120-page publication by the American Public Health Association entitled *Community Organization for*

*Health Education.* This publication was issued in 1941. It was later reprinted and its wide distribution continued.

Much was learned from this study. We found that health departments, public schools, and voluntary health agencies were all involved when programs were most successful. Many of the campaigns had quite significant results. For example, Bulloch County, Georgia had a campaign for improved sanitation and the reduction of hookworm disease. A survey had shown that 60% of the schoolchildren were infested with hookworm in 1936 when the program began. By the spring of 1940, several hundred sanitary privies had been built and the incidence of hookworm among schoolchildren had been reduced to 27.7%.

In some cases the program of health education and community action was started from within the health department. In other cases action was initiated by the school system or by a voluntary agency. Both the sequence of events and the framework of community organization varied among the communities studied. Here are some of the principles which the committee reported as growing out of the study:*

1. The planning group needs to represent all the people concerned, and the discussions must include some people with a specific knowledge of health problems.
2. Leadership is needed by a person or persons in a position to work objectively with all conflicting groups, and possessing ability in group work and adult education. Such a person is likely to be at different times a stimulator, catalytic agent, educator, counsellor, and mediator.
3. The technique of asking questions is often important in developing community organization and group discussion.
4. It is always important to consider into what hands power is being given to make decisions. Usually major decisions should remain with the entire group.

*From "Health Education and Community Organization," *Journal of School Health,* Oct.-Nov. 1949, a paper which had been read by C. E. Turner before the Public Health Education Section of the American Public Health Association.

5. There is no single best plan for community organization. Local factors and available personnel will determine the type of organization.

6. In successful joint programs, persons and organizations have subordinated their individual desires and interests to the purpose of the joint project. Even though some individuals or groups must play more important parts than others, a dominating attitude cannot be assumed if the program is to succeed.

7. When the joint-committee type of action is used, those agreeing to the plans should make no mental reservations about their agreement.

8. If the plan for cooperation is well made, it sets up good administrative procedures. It defines the functions of agencies and of staff members. This facilitates joint relationships. If the mechanism of cooperation does not do these things, friction ensues which may disrupt the harmony of the program.

9. While the mechanism of cooperation is important, the people who operate it are even more so. A good mechanical plan can succeed only when the people who operate it are broad enough to see its values, are compatible personally, and are not antagonistic professionally.

Community organization for health education has been reflected in many community campaigns. Health promotion and cooperation in health education has taken place at the state level and the national level. We had a very successful local campaign against poison oak in Berkeley, California in 1946-47, carried out by students in my class in health education in the School of Public Health. I will tell you about it some time.

# 25

## IRAN AND O.C.I.

On Friday, December 10, 1948, I was visiting the State Offices of the National Foundation for Infantile Paralysis in Columbus, Ohio, when the secretary said Boston was trying to reach me on the telephone. Startled by the possibility that there might be sickness at home, I hastened to the phone to find that the call was from Professor Moreland of M.I.T., a member of the firm of Jackson & Moreland, Engineers. He said his firm was one of a group forming Overseas Consultants, Inc. (OCI)*, which had been engaged by Iran to study various phases of national life and recommend a program of development for the country over a seven-year period. He invited me to go to Iran as the public health expert with that group of specialists.

Both my wife and Mr. O'Connor reacted favorably to my going and on Friday, January 21, 1949 four of us (the spe-

*OCI was composed of the American Appraisal Company; Coverdale & Colpitts; Ebasco Services, Incorporated; Ford, Bacon and Davis, Incorporated; Jackson & Moreland; Madigan-Hyland; F. H. McGraw & Company; Sanderson & Porter; Standard Research Consultants, Incorporated; Stone & Webster Engineering Corporation; and the J. G. White Engineering Corporation.

The following list of topics covered in its report indicates the kinds of experts employed in the Iran study (we numbered some thirty persons, although we were not all in Iran at the same time): Public Health, Education, Agriculture, Water Resources, Meteorology, Surveying and Mapping, Town Improvement and Housing, Transportation, Communications, Industry and Mining, Electric Power, Petroleum, Statistical Organization, Distribution, Legal Matters and Economic Problems. The five-volume printed report of 1064 pages plus over 100 pages of charts and other exhibits was submitted to the government of Iran late in 1949. Since OCI was employed under a contractual arrangement, the report was not distributed outside the Iranian government.

cialist in international education, a secretary, the office manager, and myself) started our flight to Iran as the first contingent of the OCI staff. Other specialists soon began arriving in Teheran. I was employed on this project until April 24. OCI was an example of the remarkable efficiency of private industry. It was thrilling for all of us to be asked by the "King of Kings" to study his country and suggest the ways in which the government should move in the proposed Seven-Year Development Plan.

In the month between my contract and my departure, evenings and Sundays were given to reading about Iran. A book which had just come out was especially helpful *(Iran, Past and Present,* by D. N. Wilber, Princeton University Press, 1948). I talked with OCI leadership, with our contact in the U.S. State Department, and with Mr. Nemazi, who had recently established the Iran Foundation. I learned, for example, that "Iran" (meaning "bridge") is to be used, not Persia (from Persis, the sub-kingdom from which came Cyrus, who overthrew the Median ruler in 553 B.C. and went on to establish the first world empire). The country is nearly the size of the United States east of the Mississippi. It had a population just under 17,000,000 people, only about 3,000,000 of whom lived in towns of more than 20,000 inhabitants. About two million belonged to nomadic tribes.

The Pahlavi dynasty was established in 1925 when a special Constituent Assembly acclaimed Reza Kahn as Shahinshah. His son, Muhammad Reza Shah Pahlavi, ascended to the throne in 1941. Ninety-eight percent of the inhabitants are Moslems.

There are ten *ostans* or provinces. Teheran, the capital, with its 750,000 people, had *quanats* or unique underground channels bringing water from the snow-covered mountain peaks, and *jubes* or open drainage ditches. But it also had its palaces, its collection of precious stones in support of the currency, its Institute of Ancient Persian Arts, and its Majlis or parliament.

The four of us arrived in the snow of winter and the

clear, crisp air of the high elevation of Teheran. We were established in a big house still higher than the city—although later, when our staff became larger, we rented a new house and established our own menage in town. As we began meeting government officials it did not seem like being in a foreign country. This was partly because most of the men we met spoke English—and always without an accent—and because of the spirit of hospitality.

Iranian hospitality is indeed something to note. One day when walking along outside a village, I saw three laborers having their lunch of bread and cheese beside the road. They saw me coming, and one got up and offered me some of their lunch. Where in America would workmen offer to share their lunch with a foreign passerby?

The first day I visited a village I was invited to see the baking of bread in a circular iron cylinder inside of which a fire of small twigs had been built. The dough was made into a flat "pancake" shape and stuck on the outside of the cylinder to cook. When it was done, the woman, apparently the grandmother of the family, took off and "broke" the large, round, thin piece of bread, offering me a piece. Although I was not hungry, I, of course, accepted the opportunity to break bread with the family. If one is invited to a meal by a villager, the neighbors secretly bring bits of food to the kitchen of the host in order that the hospitality of the village may be of high order.

One of my most happy experiences was a luncheon given to three of us by the Gashgai brothers, the heads of their tribe, in Shiraz. Following lunch, two of us drove on south and stopped for supper with the Sheik in a mountain village.

What a gracious host! We sat on the ground in a part of the huge tent separated by a black blanket from the rest of the household and its activities. Our food was placed on a spotless cloth spread out on the earth between us.

We had eaten more than one should at a single meal when our host told us that this was an appetizer, that we would walk about the village and then come back for dinner. The walk to see the horses, choice goats and camels, the long strip of Persian rug being made by the women, and the general layout of the village, was most interesting; but the excess of delicious food when we returned to the tent was overpowering. The conversation with our host, through interpretation, dealt with many phases of Iranian life. It included the following exchange directly related to hospitality.

"You will have the tent just in front of this one for the night," said the host.

"I am sorry we cannot stay," I replied. "We have to go to Bushire tonight."

"I have soldiers enough to detain you," said he.

"I am sure you do," I replied. "The next time I come to Iran I will come back to your village and stay so long you will want me to go away."

"I shall have soldiers enough to send you away," said the Sheik. "But you see my difficulty. Always I have military superiority but always I am defeated because you are the guest."

My first days in Iran brought many contacts with leaders of government and of voluntary, religious, and social agencies. An early contact was with an American named Noe (a young graduate of the School of Public Health of the University of North Carolina) who was a representative of the American Near East Foundation, directing a remarkable program of village improvement in the Veramine plain. He introduced me to Dr. A. Torab Mehra, whom we invited to join us on a trip to Isfahan, Shiraz and Bushire covering the period of February 10 to 20.

Dr. Mehra had recently returned to his native land as Medical Director of the Iran Foundation following his M.D. and M.P.H. degrees in the United States. His wife is an American. His knowledge of Iran, his American training, and his remarkable ability gave him much to contribute to a public health survey of Iran. Upon our return to Teheran I asked him whether there was any possibility of arranging for him to give some time to our project. He cabled the headquarters of the Iran Foundation in New York, and the next day he had a return cable instructing him to give all his time to Professor Turner so long as he could be useful. He worked with me throughout my stay to our mutual satisfaction.

Some help in special investigations was also secured from staff members of the Ministry of Health and some of the voluntary agencies. The survey included detailed investigation of existing health conditions with reference to morbidity and mortality, and a study of environmental sanitation plus an examination of all existing health activities. A recommended public health program was proposed upon the basis of these findings.

There were innumerable fascinating experiences. Three of us spent a morning in conference with Her Royal Highness, Princess Ashraf, twin sister of the Shah and President of the Imperial Organization for Social Service.

At one time Dr. Mehra and I drove along the Caspian to Resht, where the Provincial Health Officer said, "Oh, yes, I heard on the Russian radio that a Dr. Turner was coming here. They said he is really an army general in the guise of a public health expert."

One day we had for lunch caviar which had been taken from the fish that morning. On an auto trip to the Persian Gulf we passed over the remarkable highway built by the Allies and used for the transportation of 400,000 tons of war materials to the Russians in World War II.

A visit to the public bath of a village showed a unique type of institution. Much of the building was under ground and the water in the big cement tank was kept warm by a fire underneath attended by an old man who gave his full time to the occupation. Inside the building beside the tank were places where the bathers could rest and dry themselves and separate stalls where they could leave their clothes. The women used the bath in the afternoon when the men were at work. The men used the bath in the evening.

On my visit to an abattoir in the study of food sanitation

a touching scene was observed. From a balcony I looked down into the yards through which animals passed to the slaughterhouse. Just inside the outer gate sat a small boy about six years of age with his arms around the neck of a goat, which must have been his special pet. He would talk to the goat and pat it in the most loving fashion. The explanation of this situation seemed quite apparent. The family had found it necessary to sell the goat, and the lad was staying with his pet until the last possible moment.

Our life in the OCI house was friendly and enjoyable. Our servants had served in Iranian homes and, try as we might, we could not get them to prepare dinner before 8:30. We soon learned to use the time between work and dinner for exchanging professional experiences and nibbling pistachio nuts, caviar and crackers (a drinking-glass full of caviar cost about 75 cents). It was a time for such good-natured banter as is reflected in the following story.

One day Dr. Mehra said that the Iran-American Society was having a supper party with bridge and dancing, and that Mrs. Mehra had arranged for a friend of hers to join the three of us for both the cards and the dancing. The day after the party the gang felt like "putting me on."

"Did you see Professor Turner at the party?" said one.

"Yes, he was dancing with a beautiful Persian lady," said another, "but he did not introduce us to her."

I told them I hoped they did not expect me to find a Persian lamb and throw her to the American wolves.

Some of the most thrilling of our experiences came at No Ruz, the Persian New Year, which occurs on March 21, the first day of spring and the sun's vernal equinox. It begins five days of official holidays devoted to social calls. Houses are decorated; everyone dresses up; minor governmental employees and household servants get an extra month's wages. The folks in the villages come to see their relatives in the cities; and it seemed like the folks in the city know they are coming so they all go to the country.

No Persian, from the office cleaning help to the ministers,

worked during No Ruz, so our group planned a seminar on Iran. Each specialist was given a half-day in which to explain the problems of the country in his area of interest, give suggestions as to their solution, and answer questions and challenges from the group. Can you imagine anything more interesting than participating in such discussions of education, health, forests, agriculture, oil, water resources, transportation, communications, industry, mining, and electric power?

By mid-April the report was finished, but by then we had heard that two men in Iran had each prepared proposed public health programs for the 7-Year Plan; and it seemed likely that the one thing upon which they would agree was that the OCI plan would be worse than either of theirs. Our procedure in getting consideration and acceptance of the OCI plan was as follows.

The younger brother of the Shah, a recent graduate of Harvard and Honorary Head of the Seven-Year Plan, granted me a long interview and said he would support my request for a conference with the national leaders most directly concerned with public health. I then took the proposal to the official head of the plan. He said, "We do not put our feet under the same table with our political opponents, and the people on your list will not meet together."

He did agree, however, to translate the invitation into Persian. When it was ready I went to his office and asked whether I might deliver each invitation personally instead of having them mailed. To this he agreed. I went first to the Medical Director of the Social Service Organization. He said, "These men will not come to your meeting." But he himself agreed to come. The others did the same, and on a Tuesday morning the conference started with the key persons from the Ministry of Health, the Imperial Organization for Social Service, the Army Medical Corps, the Red Lion and Sun, the Medical School of the University of Teheran, the Iran Foundation, the Near East Foundation, and the Rockefeller Foundation.

Some of the group spoke only English and some only Persian; but several were bi-lingual. Seating was arranged so that each bi-lingual person had an English-speaking person on one side and a Persian-speaking person on the other. Thus the meeting could be conducted with universal participation by the medium of whispered translations.

We began by agreeing to make a list of all the public health activities which might be considered in planning a health program. There were some tight moments at first; but this topic was not controversial, and by the end of the day we were rolling along pretty well.

The next question was, "What should be the basis of determining priorities?" This also was not controversial; and the longer we worked together the more fun it was. Next we set out to choose the "number one" problem. Fortunately for the discussion, malaria was so severe that everyone agreed it should have first priority.

We went on from there. At no time did either Dr. Mehra or I mention our plan or what we proposed. We proceeded from question to question and made clear notes of our agreements.

When Thursday night came we had not finished. Friday is the Holy Day. Everyone agreed to return on Saturday. By noon Saturday we had finished four days of most constructive planning in which practically complete agreement had been reached upon a program which differed in no essential way from the "report" Dr. Mehra and I had prepared.

The next step was to announce the plan with credit to the distinguished Iranians who had participated in the conference. This was done in a press release that afternoon.

The general framework of the health survey and the scope of the recommendations in the 77 printed pages of the OCI public health report are seen in the following abbreviated outline:

I. Present Health Conditions with respect to
   A. Mortality and Morbidity

1. Communicable Disease preventable through (1) insect control, (2) sanitation, (3) limiting contacts with infected persons, (4) immunization and (5) good obstetrical and infant care.
2. Non-Communicable Diseases

B. Environmental Sanitation in respect to insects which transmit disease, excreta disposal, water supply, ice, milk and food, housing, baths, school sanitation, industrial sanitation, garbage and rubbish disposal.

II. Present Health Activities of Official Agencies and Voluntary Agencies.

III. Proposed Public Health Program with reference to malaria prevention, general sanitation, public health education, public health laboratories, tuberculosis, syphilis, trachoma, vaccination, maternal and child health, industrial hygiene, school hygiene, quarantine, National Institute of Health, drug addiction, mental hygiene, dental hygiene, vital statistics, nutrition survey, recreational survey, manufacture of antibiotics, rural health program, personnel training, and administrative costs (overall budget).

Much of the program proposed by OCI was delayed for a few years because difficulties arose at that time between the Iranian Government and the Anglo-Iranian Oil Company, temporarily cutting off a major source of income. This delay did not hit the public health program, however. Acting upon the recommendations that malaria should receive first attention, over 1,000 villages were sprayed with DDT the next summer; and the sudden absence of mosquitoes and the sharp reduction in malaria produced a demand from the people and an eagerness on the part of the government to continue public health activities. Collaboration from WHO, the Iran Foundation, the Rockefeller Foundation, and other agencies has assisted in the development of an extensive public health program which has been a significant element in the remarkable progress of Iran in the last twenty years. A return visit to the country for WHO and Unesco in 1962, and a visit on my own in 1966, revealed an excellent Ministry of Health, the sound activities of voluntary health agencies, and the continued hospitality and charm so characteristic of the Iranian people.

*Note:* The following statement summarizing health conditions is taken from the thesis of Dr. Mehra presented to the School of Public Health of John Hopkins University in 1969:

> The first comprehensive report on health characteristics of Iran was prepared in 1949 by Professor Clair E. Turner. A summary of Dr. Turner's observations in 1949 was as follows:
>
> 1. Among the insect-borne diseases, malaria, with an estimated three million to five million cases annually, is a principal national health problem. Typhus fever epidemics are common and leishmaniasis is widespread.
>
> 2. Among diseases preventable through general sanitation, diarrhea is an important cause of the high infant death rate, which is estimated at over 500 per 1,000 live births. Ascariasis, typhoid fever, para-typhoid fever, the dysenteries, and food infections are widespread. Anthrax, brucellosis, bovine tuberculosis and tapeworm infections are problems of importance.
>
> 3. Trachoma, tuberculosis, and the venereal diseases may be grouped with malaria and the intestinal diseases as the foremost national health problems. Pediculosis, scabies and fungus diseases of the scalp are widespread. The common infectious diseases of children are generally distributed throughout the country, and there are at least 7,000 cases of leprosy.
>
> 4. Those diseases which are preventable through immunization (smallpox, typhoid fever, typhus fever, diphtheria, scarlet fever, whooping cough and tetanus) are also common and widespread. The absence of ob-

stetrical and midwifery service in most of the country results in many maternal deaths from puerperal infections and from hemorrhage, and in deaths among the newborn.

5. We are without data on non-communicable diseases such as cancer, diseases of the heart and blood vessels, diabetes and nephritis. All of the dietary deficiency diseases are to be found in Iran, but their extent is unknown, as is also the extent of mental diseases and dental ailments. It is estimated that there are over 1,000,000 opium addicts.

6. There is no adequate program of insect control, and cities and towns are still without sanitary water supplies and without sewerage systems. Ice is made in the cities from polluted water and distributed without adequate sanitary precautions. The spread of disease through milk is restricted only by the general custom of using boiled and soured milk. Food is neither dispensed nor kept under sanitary conditions. Housing for the poor is crowded, inadequate, and unsanitary, and village baths spread infections. Industrial sanitation varies widely in quality, and school sanitation is generally inadequate.

Dr. Mehra's thesis goes on to indicate the great progress which has been made in the years since 1949.

# 26

## THE BEGINNING OF HEALTH EDUCATION AT W.H.O.*

It is always pleasant to participate in establishing a new and worthwhile program or activity. Mr. O'Connor had just given me permission to be absent from the National Foundation to go to Iran when I received a letter from the World Health Organization representative at the United Nations in New York. He said that the Geneva headquarters of WHO was considering the establishment of health-education activities and asked whether I would be available for six months to a year to plan the program.

I hesitated to go to Mr. O'Connor with another request for leave of absence, but he was most considerate. He said that I could not be away from the Foundation for six months at a time, but that if I would return to the Foundation in the early spring after my visit to Iran, I could go to WHO in mid-summer for two or three months.

How well things often fit together! Dr. Brock Chisholm, the Director General of WHO, invited me to stop in Geneva

*This story tells you about the beginning of the present and continuing program of health education in the World Health Organization. But the following quotation from my longhand diary in September, 1935, when Mrs. Turner and I visited Geneva, shows that some consideration had been given to health education at the time of the League of Nations:

"Geneva, September 13. Dr. Boudreau met us. Visited Assembly of the League and heard Laval, Aga Khan and others. Visited Health Section of the League.

"September 14. Heard Litvinov and others at League. Met Bonnet, who will consider health education as a cooperative activity for his Section and the Health Section of the League and will see Dr. Boudreau about it before he leaves Geneva."

on my way home from Iran. This I did, April 20 and 21, 1949. The visit was especially helpful in making WHO contacts because Dr. Chisholm invited me to discuss the proposed public health program for Iran before his Technical Planning Committee, consisting of the heads of several WHO divisions. They were pleased with the plans for Iran and, since health education was a new activity to most of them, I probably had a more favorable first contact with them as a public health expert than I would have had as a health educator. I had long discussions with the Director General concerning the philosophy of health education, and he asked me to seek and recommend to him a suitable person to head up WHO's health education activities.

Following my return to the office of the National Foundation in New York, the search for WHO's health educator began. Inquiry was made concerning the outstanding and best-trained public health educators, which resulted in the selection of A. Helen Martikainen, who had received her graduate professional education at Yale and had had most successful experiences in North Carolina and other places.

The Turners returned to Geneva the first week in July as a family. Dr. Grzegorzewski had rented us his apartment for two months while his family was away from Geneva on vacation. He had also given us wise advice as to the kind of automobile we should purchase to bring with us. He said that American cars whose top could be easily raised to allow sight-seeing in the mountains were still scarce in Europe since the war. Consequently, we purchased a small car with a soft top which folded back upon touching a button on the dashboard. It made an ideal car for touring and sold at the end of our summer for its cost on the docks at Le Havre.

In 1949 Mary Frances was twenty and Frederick was ten, making a delightful and compact family for week-end tourism from Friday afternoons to Sunday evening or Monday morning.

Some of these week-end trips were especially interesting. For example, the trip to St. Bernard Pass allowed us to look into Italy and see the home of the St. Bernard dog. We were disappointed to find that the dogs at the monastery were less beautiful than the prize specimens we had seen at the American dog shows.

And then there was the trip where we were dangerously near falling over a precipice. Looking at the road map in the office, my secretary suggested the shortest road to the village where we were going. She said that the road was not used much, but afterward we found that it had been actually condemned for tourist travel. Going down carefully on the edge of the mountain, we met a passenger bus coming toward us. They were on the inside and we inched by them most dangerously. Frederick said, "When I get back to school this fall I will write a story called 'Three Inches from Death.' "

WHO in 1949 was still a relatively small organization. The friendliness and cordiality of Director General Chisholm made it a happy place to work. On the first day of my return to the WHO office (which was then in the old League of Nations Building), as I stood in line in the cafeteria, someone touched my elbow. I looked around and saw that it was the Director General with a cordial welcome-back greeting. This was typical of him and typical of the optimism and cordiality which characterized the new international organization.

There was good luck on the professional side. Dr. Martha Eliot had been brought to Geneva as Assistant Director General. Her interest in health education made it possible to move rapidly and bring Miss Martikainen to Geneva in mid-September.

On September 1, the Grzegorzewskis came back to their apartment. Mrs. Turner and the children returned home, and my schedule for the first part of September was to visit public health and education authorities in European countries. September 6 to 10 were given over in Paris to visits to Unesco and the Ministry of Health. From September 11 to 14, I was in London, 15 to 17 in Frankfurt, 18 to 20 in The Hague. These visits developed professional contacts for the new unit called "Health Education of the Public" and indicated to the countries visited the kind of cooperation and assistance which would be available. The last ten days of September were spent in joint planning with Miss Martikainen in setting up plans for health education representation in the six regions of WHO and plans for the activities in the headquarters office.

My relationships with health education in WHO have continued ever since its establishment. They have involved membership in the Expert Advisory Panel of the Health Education Section, serving as Consultant to Expert Committees, secondment to Unesco for health education services in Egypt* and Iraq, a study leading to a publication, *Planning for Health Education in Schools,* which is now in nine languages, and service as Chief of Health Education for the period 1962 to 1964 while Miss Martikainen was away on study leave for her doctorate.

Almost everyone has heard the internationally-used WHO definition of health as "a state of complete physical, mental and social well-being, not merely the absence of disease or infirmity." I had often wondered when and from whom it came. On a visit to WHO in April 1961, I asked the secretary in the Director General's office who could help me find out. I was referred to the librarian, Mr. H. A. Izant. He said, "You are very lucky. Mr. Howard B. Calderwood is visiting us this

---

*Readers who have served abroad may be interested in the following incident. Senousi Rashdan, my sightseeing guide in Cairo, who had been to Mecca as a pilgrim and had very interesting acquaintances, took me to meet a friend who was an archaeologist and a dealer in rare antiques. His friend said, "I saw your picture in the daily paper yesterday taken with the Minister of Education. The paper said you are living and working in one of the little villages a few miles from Cairo."

Later in the visit when I was looking at a scarab ring; I said, "How much is this ring?"

"Nothing," he replied.

"What do you mean?" said I.

"I mean that you are to take the ring and pay me nothing," he replied. "If you are willing to leave a comfortable life in America and come to work in that dirty village, you must take home something to prove that at least one Egyptian appreciates what you are doing."

week and I will take you to him. He was an advisor to the U.S. State Department and served as Secretary of the Technical Preparatory Committee for the Health Conference held in Paris 18 March to 5 April, 1946."

Mr. Izant did take me to Mr. Calderwood, from whom I secured the following information.

The minutes of the Technical Preparatory Committee meeting for 20 March contain a statement by Dr. Brock Chisholm concerning the task ahead to the effect that the Committee "should do their utmost to bring all the peoples of the world together in the service of physical, social and emotional health."

On 21 March, 1946 a Sub-Committee on the Preamble consisting of Dr. S. Sze, Chairman, Dr. G. Bermann, Dr. Brock Chisholm and Dr. J. Cancik, submitted a "Draft of Preamble to the Convention of the World Health Organization," the first paragraphs of Annex 10 being as follows:

"The States parties to this World Convention recognize these fundamental truths, which are deemed to be basic to the acceptable interrelationship of all peoples in a world at peace.

"The right to health is one of the fundamental rights to which every human being, without distinction of race, sex, language or religion, is entitled.

"Health is not only the absence of infirmity or disease but also a state of physical fitness and mental and social well-being."

The last paragraph of Annex 10 stated:

"The States parties to the World Convention, recognizing these truths, hereby establish as a specialized agency the World Health Organization, through which nations will cooperate for the protection and promotion of health throughout the world."

Thus the WHO definition of health appears to have arisen from group thinking and agreement; but the contribution of Dr. Brock Chisholm to the shaping of that definition was obviously a major one.

# 27

## THE FOUNDING OF THE SOCIETY OF PUBLIC HEALTH EDUCATORS

The oldest health education association of any kind is, I believe, the New England Health Education Association which was organized by the 1925 summer school class in health education at M.I.T. and is thus approaching its 50th year. It has become a thriving organization contributing to health education in both school and extra-school programs.

The initiation of activities looking toward the establishment of the first national society of public health educators made up of practicing health education specialists came in the nineteen forties from Dr. Lucy S. Morgan and her colleagues on the faculty of the University of North Carolina. By that time various health education organizations existed, but they were open to anyone interested in health education. Professional education for health educators had been spreading and increasing in volume since the first course offered in the Harvard-MIT School of Public Health in 1921-22. It is not strange that within a quarter century there should develop a desire for a society made up of graduate and experienced full-time specialists in public health education.

Dr. Morgan already had a splendid program of graduate study in operation at North Carolina University, and it was a natural place for such a movement to get underway. Fortunately for the historical record, her colleague, Dr. Eunice N. Tyler, prepared an excellent statement of the step-by-step developments for the first annual report of the Society issued in 1951,* from which she has given me permission to quote.

*Tyler, Eunice N., A New Profession Comes of Age; in the report entitled Organization and First Annual Meeting, 1950-51, and published by the Society of Public Health Educators.

As Dr. Tyler pointed out, there were an estimated 460 health educators employed by official and voluntary health agencies in 1947. Her report continues:

"The first concrete step toward organization was taken in March 1948 at the Third Annual Working Conference for Health Education Alumni held at the School of Public Health in Chapel Hill, North Carolina. The fifty-six participants, who were from fourteen states, were emphatic about the need for organization, but reminded themselves that they were not a representative group. They decided to go home and talk the matter over with as many health educators as possible. They also voted to promote further discussion at the Annual Meeting of the Southern Branch of the American Public Health Association to be held in New Orleans in early April, and elected the writer as temporary chairman, responsible for calling the meeting.

"On April 13, 1948, public health educators from eight southern states gathered at a special meeting in New Orleans and Miss A. Helen Martikainen served as secretary. This group concluded, as had those at the earlier conference at Chapel Hill, that organization was desirable, but that health educators from other sections of the country should have an opportunity to express their views. Several methods were selected for involving more persons. Dr. Lucy S. Morgan was asked to discuss the proposal with health educators in Colorado, California, and Arkansas, since she expected to be in those states within a few weeks. Each person present agreed to contact all the health educators he knew throughout the country, and ask them to send their suggestions to the Temporary Chairman. . . .

"During the Annual Meeting of the American Public Health Association in Boston in October 1948, two more informal meetings were held. The first included as many State Chairmen and other public health educators as could be rounded up on short notice. Stress was again put on the need for much wider participation, and two important decisions were made—first, to hold an open meeting during the convention to introduce the idea of a professional organization to all health educators who cared to attend and give them a chance to express their opinions, and second, to invite a group of leaders in the field from the United States, Canada, and Puerto Rico to serve as a Temporary Steering Committee to explore the idea further.

"Discussion in the second Boston meeting centered chiefly around possible objectives. . . . Several participants helped define health educa*tion* as one of the many responsibilities of all persons in the field of health, and the health educa*tor* as the specially-trained worker who could take major responsibility and serve as a resource person to other health workers. . . .

"During December 1948, in line with the Boston recommendations, a number of health education leaders from the United States, Canada, and Puerto Rico were asked to join the small informal group that had been studying the proposal for a professional organization. Together they formed a Temporary Steering Committee, composed of the following members:

Mr. Gordon Bunch, S. C.
Mr. Homer N. Calver, N. Y.
Dr. Mayhew Derryberry, D.C.
Miss Vivian V. Drenckhahn, N. Y.
Miss Mary Catherine Drennan, Fla.
Dr. Ruth E. Grout, Minn.
Mrs. Ann W. Haynes, Calif.
Dr. Ira V. Hiscock, Conn.
Miss Sally Lucas Jean, N. Y.
Mrs. Alice M. Johnson, D.C.
Miss Mary Lou King, Tex.
Mr. Milton E. Kossack, La.
Dr. Granville W. Larimore, N. Y.
Mr. Sol S. Lifson, N. Y.
Dr. Howard W. Lundy, Wash.
Miss A. Helen Martikainen, N. C.

Miss Helen Massengale, Tenn.
Dr. Lucy S. Morgan, N. C.
Mr. B. T. McMillon, N. C.
Mr. J. Louis Neff, Tex.
Miss Margaret E. Nix, Canada
Dr. Dorothy B. Nyswander, Calif.
Mrs. Mary H. Parks, N. Y.
Miss Beryl J. Roberts, Mass.
Miss Lucretia Ann Saunders, Calif.
Mrs. Rae K. Shoemaker, N. Y.
Miss Cassie B. Smith, Miss.
Dr. Warren H. Southworth, Wisc.
Dr. Helen M. Starr, Minn.
Dr. Ruth Sumner, Ga.
Dr. Clair E. Turner, N. Y.
Dr. Eunice N. Tyler, N. C.
Miss Maria Varela, Puerto Rico

"In June 1949, the writer, who had served as Temporary Chairman for fifteen months, asked to be relieved of this responsibility, and Dr. Clair E. Turner agreed to take over the chairmanship. . . .

"A real milestone was reached when representatives of the Temporary Steering Committee met in New York on October 21 and 22, 1949, immediately prior to the Annual Meeting of the American Public Health Association. . . . On the afternoon of October 22 the Temporary Steering Committee adjourned, and reconvened as the Society of Public Health Educators, Interim Commission."

The Interim Commission and its committees worked industriously on problems of organization; and by the time of the St. Louis meeting of the American Public Health Association, the group was ready for definite action. The organization of the society took place on October 27 and 28, 1950. Its first officers were:

President: Dr. Clair E. Turner
President-Elect: Dr. Mayhew Derryberry

Vice-President: Mr. Levitte B. Mendel
Secretary: Mr. J. Louis Neff
Treasurer: Dr. Ruth E. Grout

The criteria for membership were reflected in the following quote from Article III of the Constitution:

> The following shall be eligible for election as active fellows:
>
> a) A person who has a graduate degree with a major or specialization in health education, accredited by this Society, and who has had at least two years of experience in health education.
>
> b) A person holding a bachelor's or professional degree involving training in education, basic sciences or social sciences;
>
> and
>
> Who has been actively engaged as a public health educator on a full-time basis for at least five years;
>
> and
>
> Who is now responsible for the professional direction of, supervision of, or consultation to important public health education work on the local, state or national level in:
>
> aa. An official health agency
>
> or
>
> bb. A voluntary health agency
>
> or
>
> cc. Other organization engaged in a significant overall public health education program.
>
> c) A full-time teacher of professional rank in an institution of higher learning preparing for degrees accredited by this Society. . . .
>
> d) Other individuals who have made an outstanding contribution in the field of public health education may be invited to become fellows of the Society.

You may have noted that membership was directed primarily toward health educators employed by official or voluntary health agencies. However, a committee was created at the St. Louis meeting to "seek ways of strengthening relationships between public health education and school health education."

In 1951 the society had 60 members. In 1972 it had over 700 members.

# 28

# THE INTERNATIONAL UNION FOR HEALTH EDUCATION

The first international non-governmental agency in health education was the International Union for Health Education. It was conceived and proposed in France by Professor Jacques Parisot and Mr. Lucien Viborel.

Dr. Parisot was Professor of Public Health in the Medical School at Nancy, and a public health statesman of note, having served as President of the WHO Assembly, as well as having given leadership to public health in France. At the time the Union was founded he was Chairman of the Executive Council of the World Health Organization.

The other man, Lucien Viborel, was one of the most experienced health educators in Europe and a man of charming personality, international spirit and great vision. At the time of the founding of the union he was Director of the National Center for Health Education in the Ministry of Public Health of France. His work in health education began with the national anti-tuberculosis program of France which followed World War I.

Under stimulation from Professor Parisot and Mr. Viborel, the French Government promoted the organization of the Constitutive Assembly of the union in May, 1951, at an international conference in Paris. Letters of invitation to this conference were sent to the various countries of the world and to international organizations. More than fifty countries and twenty international organizations were represented by delegates. WHO and Unesco sent observers.

It happened that I was in Geneva at the time of the meeting, on my way back home from a WHO-Unesco assignment in Egypt and Iraq. The Director General asked me to join Dr. Grzegorzewski, chief of the WHO program in professional education and fellowships, and Miss Martikainen, chief of Health Education, in representing WHO at the meeting.

Mr. Viborel and I had become acquainted during my visit to Paris in September 1949. I found at that visit that I had already had indirect contact with him. You can imagine my surprise when, upon entering his office, I saw on the wall back of his desk a large picture of Professor Selskar Gunn who was my predecessor on the teaching staff at M.I.T. Mr. Viborel's contact with him dated back to the end of World War I. At that time France was suffering heavily from tuberculosis. The Rockefeller Foundation made a grant for fighting the disease, and Professor Gunn and Dr. Lindley Williams were sent over to direct the program. Mr. Viborel had just finished the university and was placed in charge of one of the traveling equips which moved about the country doing education against tuberculosis. He had continued in health education from that time.

I had never met Professor Parisot until the morning of the meetings when he came over to me to ask in French whether I thought such a union could be of value. I told him, "Yes," and he said, "I think Mr. Viborel should be Secretary of the group." I agreed, and he continued, "And you should be the President."

"Me?" I asked in astonishment. "I must decline. I am here merely as an observer for WHO."

After the morning session, Dr. Grzegorzewski, Miss Martikainen and I got together to discuss WHO relationships, and I told them of Professor Parisot's proposal, explaining that refusal of the honor seemed proper because I was not an official representative of the Society of Public Health Educators or any other voluntary group in America. Their point of view was quite different. They felt it was important for the proposed union to be closely related to health education in WHO. I could provide such a relationship but neither of them could do so because such non-governmental activities were prohibited to staff members of the World Health Organization. I yielded to this advice although I feared some unfavorable reaction from health educators in the U.S.A. for doing so.

The organizing group took the form of an interim commission for which I served as Chairman. Two years later the formal organization took place at the 1953 meeting in Paris with Professor Parisot as the Honorary President of the Union, Mr. Viborel as the Secretary General, and myself as the first President, serving until the meeting in Rome in 1956.

The subsequent meetings—Dusseldorf in 1959 under President L'Eltore, Philadelphia in 1962 under President Canaperia, Madrid in 1965 under President Ennes, and Buenos Aires in 1959 under President Bosch Marin—have reflected in their published reports current activities and developments in health education around the world. From 1956 to 1968 I served as Chief Advisor, at which time I was named Honorary President.

Each of the world meetings has had incidental items of special interest. In Rome the organizational meeting was in a building at the head of the Appian Way, in a room which was reserved for conferences of the president of the country. He happened to be away from Rome at this time, but his wife visited the exhibit and one of the program meetings.

At Dusseldorf I remember especially the banquet with its international representation at the speakers' table, a remarkable menu and the formal entrance of uniformed waiters with the banquet room lights out temporarily and a lighted candle on each waiter's tray.

I remember that the Philadelphia meeting was in session over the 4th of July and the Union heard an address by President John F. Kennedy.

Mr. and Mrs. Viborel paid a visit of several weeks to America where he was most cordially received and where he enjoyed many professional contacts with outstanding educators and programs. I remember especially his visit to the health education program in the Malden public schools. Dr. Mary Spencer, the director of health education, had arranged a special welcoming program for him in one of the third grades. The children greeted Mr. Viborel speaking in French in unison, and reviewed for him their health education activities.

One of the most important activities of the union has been the development of the *International Journal for Health Education* by Annette Le Meitour-Kaplun, with the generous support and assistance of her husband Sioma Kaplun, the head of one of Europe's largest printing establishments. She also served as secretary of the Union for the year following the sudden death of Mr. Viborel and preceding the secretaryship of Dr. Louis-Paul Aujoulat, the present Secretary General under whose leadership there have been important developments in international cooperation in health education.

As this manuscript goes to the printer an anniversary meeting of the Union has just been held under the Presidency of Senora de Sustaita Seeber in Paris (July 8-14, 1973). Chairmen of plenary sessions for this conference included former Presidents of the Union Mr. Howard Ennes, Dr. Giovanni Canaperia, Dr. Juan Bosch-Marin, and the Vice President for North America, Mr. Sol Lifson. The new president is Professor Raoul Senault.

## 29

## PEDRO ORATA

I must tell you about my friend Pedro Orata, a most delightful man and one of the most gifted educators I have ever known. Following a brief contact at Unesco in September 1949 when I visited Unesco to establish cooperative contact in health education between WHO and Unesco, our acquaintance grew through several subsequent meetings. We met in Geneva as members of a joint expert committee where he came as Chairman of the Unesco delegation. Our longest period together was in the Philippines in 1962 after his retirement from Unesco, and when Naomi and I were on our way through the Far East in connection with the WHO-Unesco study which produced *Planning for Health Education in Schools*. But let me tell you some of the interesting facts about this man.

Pedro was born in the barrio of Bactad in Urdaneta, Pangasinan, on February 27, 1899. He says his parents had only a small farm and an old *carabao*. He told me:

"At first I was not interested in school. The fact is that I had to repeat Grade IV, and I barely passed in the third grade. After my failing, my father put me to work on the farm. He said: 'Since you obviously do not like school, I have work for you to do on the farm.' And indeed, he had! I had to wake up at five o'clock in the morning to cook breakfast and I went to bed late at night, and only after I had washed the dishes and kitchen utensils. All day long I worked on the farm—harrowing the field, pasturing the carabao and cutting grass for it, planting the rice seedbed and later on transplanting the seedlings.

"When the year was over, I was glad enough to go back to school, and since there was no Grade IV in Bactad I had to go to the village of Urdaneta, which is four kilometers from the barrio. I had to walk over mud and water during the rainy season from July to September. By that time my father could afford to buy me a pair of shoes. I was very careful with them. When I reached a muddy place I took off my shoes and carried them over my shoulders. To economize, my father bought me a pair that was one or two sizes larger, which he thought would last a year or two longer. When I complained that the shoes were loose and they hurt my toes, he made me wear the right shoe on the left foot and the left shoe on the right foot. I confess that the arrangement felt all right even though I could not help noticing that my classmates made fun of me, which I did not mind, or minded less than the hurt on my toes.

"I must have done well enough in my second attempt in Grade IV. My teacher, who was very strict, was only a Grade IV graduate himself, but he was a good disciplinarian. Corporal punishment was not prohibited then, but I did not receive as much beating as some of my classmates. He was at the same time principal of the school. My fear of him and my recollection of the hard work on the farm made me study very hard. As a result, I began to like school better and my grades improved, but not much.

"It would have been impossible for me to continue in high school in Lingayen had not my sister, who, herself, had completed the fourth grade in Bactad, volunteered to help me. She stopped going to school and took boarders in Lingayen while I continued my studies."

When he finished high school, his sister said, "Pedro, you must go to college. Have you ever thought of going to America?"

Pedro told me he replied, "Yes, but I cannot swim that far."

He did come across the Pacific on a steerage ticket which his sister bought with money she had saved. Landing in

Seattle, he got a job with a railroad gang which was employed to keep the tracks in shape.

The gang boss was a very rough man whose speech was loaded with the heaviest profanity. These words were new to Pedro, for whom English was a third language after the native village language and Spanish. He said to himself that that was apparently the way in which English should be spoken, and he applied himself vigorously to learning that kind of English.

Following some months working on the railroad, he went to the University of Illinois where he earned his way, taking the Bachelor's and Master's degree. He recounts his first contact with the dean.

"After talking with me a bit, he said: 'Now, tell me why you use such terrible language. This is a university, you know, and not a penitentiary.' So, I told him my story—that 'In the Philippines I learned to diagram and to speak well-constructed sentences which I did not understand, but when I heard our boss speak English so meaningfully, I thought my American teachers in the Philippines had taught me the wrong English. So, I decided to change.' The old gentleman had such a good laugh listening to me that he said at the end of our conversation, 'Well, young man, how about coming home for chicken dinner next Sunday? I want my wife to listen to your story and have as good a laugh as I have just had.' "

He took his Ph.D. at Ohio State University, returning to the Philippines in 1927, where he taught in a normal school and served as a division superintendent of schools. In 1934 he returned to the United States as a member of the faculty at Ohio State University, and after two years was called to establish the first community school in the United States in the Indian reservation of Kyle, South Dakota.

In 1937 he joined the United States Office of Education. In 1941 he joined the National Council of Education, and in 1948 became a member of the staff of Unesco in Paris, where he remained until 1960. His family consisted of himself, his wife Pilar, and a very remarkable cat named Fifi. I mention Fifi because she really was a member of the family. When the Oratas returned to the Philippines upon retirement, a regular passenger ticket was bought for Fifi, so she had a seat for herself in the airplane.

Pedro had a building lot in Manila and was offered a post in the teachers college. But he decided to return to his native village where he built a modern house to which he invited Naomi and me for a visit of several days. Let me tell you about that visit.

The house was truly modern in contrast with most of the houses of the village which were of traditional construction, consisting of one or two rooms raised on stilts some six or seven feet above the ground. As Pedro said, they had everything in this house that they had in their apartment in Paris: bathrooms, electric lights, hot water, a library, and all the usual household conveniences. The house, of some seven or eight rooms, was set in a lot of perhaps a half-acre and surrounded by a stone-and-concrete wall nine or ten feet high, with a heavy iron gate which allowed the passage of their automobile. The safety of the household was guarded by three or four geecse who cried loudly whenever someone came in the gate. They were alert sentries which notified the household of the arrival of any unwelcome guests without the danger of attack which watchdogs would have given. A wide variety of fruit and vegetables grew in the garden.

Pedro did accept a lectureship in the teachers college in Manila. But a most unusual and valuable contribution to society was made at Urdaneta. We saw many of these Orata-stimulated activities during our visit. Rural schools in the area were not in session, but the teachers of half a dozen such schools nearest the village came back to their one-room schools to tidy up the place, receive Dr. Orata's guest, and tell me about their program. Papaya trees had been planted on the school grounds to contribute melons to the school lunch. Excellent sanitary facilities had been provided in each of the schools.

A village cooperative had been started to develop a herd of cattle, and we met the men who were responsible for the care of the animals. A project was under way for the growth of cocoa trees. A young plant or slip could be purchased from the government, and after four or five years it would yield a crop which would help the boy who owned it to get more schooling. We visited two or three families in the traditional-type housing, and saw mats and other handwork products which the villagers were developing for outside income.

On Sunday afternoon there was an educational meeting of parents and teachers, where current school health activities were described and future plans discussed. This was followed by a very informal and friendly late-afternoon lunch out of doors.

The practical health activities for elementary school pupils in the Urdaneta schools included not only sanitation and practice in school housekeeping but also gardening in the school gardens and family gardening at home, the composting of garbage, getting rid of flies, the drainage of pools to prevent the breeding of mosquitoes and cooperative planning between school and home. These things were being done so well that the story of this program was included in the WHO-Unesco study entitled *Planning for Health Education in Schools*. The developments at Urdaneta reflected the possibilities and social achievements of a dynamic and creative individual.

Typical of Pedro's activities was bringing the telapia fish from Thailand, to the barrio of Bactad in Urdaneta. This fish had served as an important element of the food supply of the Siamese people, and Pedro encouraged the Siamese practice of developing a fishpond in each village where this vigorous and rapidly reproducing fish could be raised to add to the protein constituent of the diet. Scores of villages through the Philippines now raise telapia.

After returning home from the world tour in which Mrs. Turner and I visited Pedro, I thought about his remarkable contributions to education, and I heard of his receiving the R. M. Magsaysay Award in the field of public service on August 31, 1971. The $10,000 has been deposited as a trust fund in a bank, and the interest is being used each year for the promotion of education projects.

In a letter to Pedro early in 1972 I asked what was the secret of his development of unusual creative ability. In his reply he said, "If I succeeded at all, it is not because of any advantage on my part, inherited or otherwise. I failed twice in school and I was a drop-out and out-of-school for two years. I could not even pass the two tests for driving a car which I took in Paris after several weeks of training under a very strict teacher. It was my lone sister who helped me go to high school, by taking boarders and doing their laundry, and who saved enough during the four years—by dropping nickels and dimes in her bamboo deposit box—to buy me a steerage ticket to America. In America, like many college students, I worked six or more hours a day—washing dishes, etc.—while going to the University of Illinois and Ohio State University. So, I have nothing that the poorest and average or below-average boy (or girl) does not have, and it is for this reason that I have been very strong in advocating our self-help school projects. What I have done, if it is of any value, anyone can do as well, if not better. How? WORK HARD, LEARN TO LEARN, HELP YOURSELF AND OTHERS!"

# 30

## PRIDE AND PREJUDICE

This is the story of two international meetings which met but never functioned, although extensive plans had been made and appreciable United Nations funds were expended. They illustrate the tremendous force of man's desire for status, recognition and political power. In reading about these meetings it should be remembered that those in attendance received instructions from their governments at home and were, therefore, not completely responsible for the decisions made.

These meetings were organized to promote health and education; but politics, the desire for racial and national status, and racism set a barrier so high and cold that meetings of the ablest specialists of many countries registered a complete and perfect failure, dealt only with intolerance and adjourned without a word of joint planning for the welfare of their people.

The first of these meetings was a regional meeting of African countries during the period of my service in Geneva as Chief of Health Education for WHO. As you may know, the World Health Organization has six regions (American, European, African, Pacific, Mid-Eastern and Southeast Asian). Each region has a high degree of autonomy and the representatives of the Ministries of Health come together each year to plan budgetary and administrative procedures. These meetings set the guidelines for the regional program of the coming year.

The first meeting I am to tell you about was held in Geneva because there was no country in the African Region which would welcome delegates from all the other countries and to which all the other delegates would go. The countries in the African Region are: Burundi, Cameroon, Central African Republic, Chad, Congo (Brazzaville) Congo (Dem. Rep. of), Dahomey, Gabon, Ghana, Guinea, Ivory Coast, Kenya, Liberia, Madagascar, Malawi, Mali, Mauritania, Mauritius, Niger, Nigeria, Rwanda, Senegal, Sierra Leone, South Africa, Southern Rhodesia, Togo, Uganda, United Republic of Tanzania, Upper Volta, and Zambia.

Immediately after the opening of the first session of this planning and budget conference, representatives of black African countries announced that they would not confer with representatives of South Africa. The Director General of WHO made a statesmanlike and lucid presentation of the situation. He pointed out that the relationships between countries were matters of politics for the consideration of the United Nations, that this meeting was made up of technicians come together to plan constructive public health programs, and that failure of WHO to work effectively in Africa would cost the lives of many native African people.

The immediate reply from several black representatives was to the effect that the loss of thousands of lives of their people would not be the slightest deterrent in their determination not to take part in any meeting or conference in which South Africa participated. They must register their violent opposition to the apartheid policies of South Africa.

It was proposed that a committee be appointed to seek a solution of the problem and to report back to the conference next day. The proposal of this committee was that the conference meet in two sections. One section would include the representatives of South Africa and any other representatives who were willing to meet in this section. The other section would be made up of all the other representatives.

Black African delegates said that this proposal reflected an apartheid kind of thinking and that it was entirely unsatisfactory. Several delegates spoke in this vein. The South African delegate rose to speak, whereupon practically all the other delegates rose in a body and left the room. They never came back. That was the end of the meeting. The African countries could not plan their own program and the planning which they should have done had to be taken over by the Office of the Director General.

Apparently men cannot put aside their racial and political prejudices in the interest of education any more than they can in the interest of health promotion. My second observation of an international meeting which failed because of the emotional and psychological reactions of groups to colonial and interracial situations was at an International Conference on Education at Geneva in 1964.* As Chief of Health Education at WHO, I was sent to this conference as an observer.

This conference was called by the International Bureau of Education and Unesco. The Unesco-I.B.E. Joint Committee sent a letter of invitation to the government of each member state and ninety-three countries sent delegations numbering in total 245 persons. A careful agenda had been developed for the consideration of (1) literacy and adult education, (2) the teaching of modern language in secondary schools, and (3) brief reports by ministries of education on educational developments during the year 1963-1964. These topics for discussion were indeed pertinent to the advancement of education throughout the world, and the delegates were of distinguished competence.

Imposing indeed was the hall full of delegates as we who were observers from organizations of the United Nations System (United Nations Relief and Works Agency, United Nations Food and Agriculture Organization, International Labor Organization, World Health Organization, and International Bank for Reconstruction and Development) took our seats at the rear. We looked over the long tables, running the length of the room and the representatives of many races, nationalities and modes of dress, to the raised platform at the front. On the platform were seats for the representatives

*The official report of this Conference is Publication No. 272 of Unesco, 84 pp.

of I.B.E. and Unesco, and for the officers of the conference; and at one side there were facilities for simultaneous interpretation in English, Russian, French and Spanish. Surely the science and art of education would be advanced by their deliberations and exchange of experiences.

The meetings did indeed start impressively, at 11 A.M. on Monday, July 6, with an address of welcome by Mr. Chavanne, Chairman of the Swiss delegation, the election of officers for the conference, and scholarly addresses by Mr. Betancur-Majia, an Assistant Director General of Unesco, and by Mr. Piaget, the Director of I.B.E.

But then trouble started and the attention of the conference became absorbed by political considerations, never to return to a discussion of education. The chairman of the Nigerian delegation demanded an explanation from the conference chairman as to why Portugal (whose colonialist policies had been condemned by the 26th Conference) should have a delegation at these meetings. The chairman reported that questions of internal regulations (including membership in the conference) had been discussed by the Executive Board of Unesco and the Council of I.B.E. They had sought to distinguish clearly between questions concerning education and those which lie in the fields of politics and law. It had been agreed to postpone the consideration of internal regulations until July 17th, at the end of the present conference. The meeting adjourned at 12:35 P.M.

The plenary session reconvened at 3:15 P.M. for five minutes, during which time the chairman proposed that the conference officers meet that afternoon with the Nigerian and other African delegations to consider the problems in hand.

On Tuesday, July 7, the conference convened at 10 A.M. The chairman presented a draft resolution he had received from the African delegations demanding that Portugal be excluded from the conference. He said that he had explained to the meeting on Monday afternoon that any attempt to change the composition of the conference by excluding Portugal would be incompatible with the decisions of I.B.E.

and Unesco, which had issued the invitations; that if such a draft resolution were submitted he would be obliged to call it inadmissible; and that, if the conference refused to acknowledge his right to do this, he would be obliged, according to the custom in his country (Austria), to resign. He recalled that I.B.E. and Unesco had decided to set aside all political matters until July 17.

It was unanimously agreed that the conference adjourn until Thursday morning in order to allow the delegations to contact their respective governments and to allow meetings among the delegations seeking a solution of the problem and a way to insure the success of the conference. The meeting adjourned at 10:40 A.M.

Thirty hours later (4 P.M. on Thursday, July 9) the conference reconvened. The African Delegations presented an appeal for the exclusion of Portugal. The Latin American countries presented a draft resolution asking that, since the official delegations came simply to deal with technical problems, discussion of the political problems be postponed until the extraordinary meeting of the council, and that the committees of the conference should begin work at once. There was heated discussion. The chairman declared the African motion inadmissable. The conference rejected his ruling (by 42 votes to 32, with 7 abstentions and 11 absences) and he resigned. The conference then adourned.

It reconvened on Friday, July 10, at 10:45, under Vice-Chairman Sawaya of Lebanon. He was elected as the new chairman, and he adjourned the meeting at 11:10 A.M. until 4:00 P.M.

From 4:00 P.M. to 7:10 P.M. the conference discussed colonialism and what procedure the conference should follow.

On Saturday similar discussions continued from 10:30 A.M. until noon.

On Monday the conference met from 11:00 A.M. to 11:20 A.M. and adjourned to allow informal group meetings.

The final session began the same day at 4:15 P.M. Thus from Monday noon, July 6, until 4:15 P.M. Monday, July 13, political considerations had dominated the conference and the educational objectives had been completely neglected. This last session also was given over to the question of the adoption of the African resolution demanding the withdrawal of Portugal.

Those in favor of the draft resolution felt that it should be passed at all costs. Those opposed to the resolution were also opposed to colonialism as a political policy but pointed out that the conference was without the legal power to change the constitution under which it was convened and urged that political considerations be laid aside and that the conference, made up of distinguished educators, give its consideration to the technical problems in the agenda. The chairman read a declaration from the Portuguese Delegation. Extensive statements were presented from Unesco and I.B.E. showing why they could not recognize the validity of a decision of the conference to exclude one of its members.

Nevertheless the conference voted to consider the African resolution and the Chairman said that he must ask for a roll-call on the issue. Some 41 delegations (including all of those from the Western Hemisphere and over a dozen from Europe) left the room. The draft resolution was adopted by 43 votes with 7 abstentions.

The director of I.B.E. and the representative of Unesco pointed out that they and their colleagues (including staff) must withdraw from the conference since they could not work under illegal circumstances. The delegates who had voted for the withdrawal of Portugal had apparently planned to continue the conference; but they found it impossible to do so because they were without staff including interpreters, recorders and secretaries. The conference rose at 6:15 P.M.

Thus the Conference failed. It is not easy to estimate the cost of this futile or worse than futile activity in money and in losing the contribution which the conference might have made to education if it had been willing to leave political problems to political bodies and address itself to the technical problems in its own field of competence.

## 31

## CALIFORNIA AND POISON OAK

In the summer of 1944, as Chief Health Education Officer for the Institute of Inter-American Affairs, I was sent to the School of Public Health of the University of California to teach a group of Latin Americans, one from each country with which the United States had a cooperative health program, in their full-time study of health education. In the fall of 1945, the war in Europe being finished, I retired from IIAA (later AID) to accept a visiting professorship at Berkeley for one to three years, in order to establish a program of study in health education. It was a most pleasant year until I ran into poison oak.

Living in the house of the head of the German Department on top of a hill which overlooked Oakland, the Bay and San Francisco, led me to buy a beautiful hillside house-lot in the valley at Orinda overlooking the golf course and having an altogether beautiful view. I went to the lot one Saturday morning in February to begin clearing the land; but I never went back to it. That night I was burning up with the itch caused by urushiol, the toxic substance produced by poison ivy, poison oak and poison sumac, and causing Rhus poisoning.

My first shock came when I asked my physician for some medication to put on the skin and was advised that "early treatment by prolonged washing with alkaline soap is effective, but *only* if undertaken within a few minutes after contact. After the area reddens and begins to itch, any treatment now known will serve only to make the patient more comfortable; it will do little to hasten recovery." I was not able to go back to my classes for about three weeks, during which time I was acutely ill with swelling, extensive rash, enlarged glands, and fever from secondary infection. I was under constant medical care.

You, as a town or city dweller, have probably never had or seen a case of Rhus poisoning; but in the 1930's, with a greater proportion of the population enjoying country living, this malady was not uncommon. (C. E. Turner, "Rhus Dermatitis as a Public Health and Health Education Problem," *American Journal of Public Health,* Vol. 37, No. 1, Jan. 1947.) The U.S. Public Health Service published a nationwide study of the incidence of the disease in 38,544 people. National estimates indicated 350,000 cases per year, with approximately 600,000 days of lost time and 465,000 medical visits.

In one student-body in a locality where the plant was profusely distributed, data upon about 5,000 students for a two-year period showed 6.5 students per thousand were hospitalized yearly, for an average of 6.9 days each. In addition, 41 students per thousand sought medical aid for Rhus poisoning but did not require hospitalization. The severity of the poisoning varied widely and the individual varied in susceptibility at different times. This is due to the fact that we are dealing with allergy and desensitization rather than with permanent immunity.

The practical impossibility for highly susceptible persons to avoid repeated poisonings is due to the extreme toxicity of urushiol, 0.001 mg. of which will cause dermatitis. Thus poisoning is transmitted not only directly but also indirectly by cats, dogs, horses, and other animals which walk over the plants, or by smoke particles from burning poison oak. The presence of hundreds of acres in the Bay area upon which poison oak was growing dimmed my hopes of an outdoor life in California. The campus at the University of California supported some luxurious growths of poison oak, one of which was within a stone's throw of the entrance to the Biology Building in which our public health classes were held.

There was, however, a cheerful side to the pursuit of information about poison oak (followed by the students and myself during my absence from the class). The most cheerful development had been the discovery of the efficacy of 2,4-D (dichlorophenoxyacetic acid), a hormone-like chemical which, in small quantities, stimulates growth but kills active broad-leaved plants completely when applied to the leaves in greater concentration. The availability of this substance obviously suggested the possibility of a community campaign in Berkeley for the eradication or reduction of poison oak.

I suggested this possibility to the health-education class, asking them whether they would prefer to do a theoretical campaign or an actual campaign. The majority of the class preferred an actual campaign, and we made plans for such a procedure. (This campaign is described in some detail in my book called "CHECK" or *Communnity Health Educators' Compendium of Knowledge,* pp. 109 to 126.)

The campaign involved (1) an investigation of the literature and the production of "Facts about Poison Oak," (2) correspondence with authorities in the field, (3) the investigation of student hospital records, (4) conferences with health, medical and recreational authorities, (5) class agreement on the basic plan, and (6) the assignment of campaign activities to individual students. One or more students were assigned to work with each of the following groups or agencies: (1) medical profession, including University of California Medical Service, (2) health department, (3) dentists, (4) nursing profession, (5) schools, (6) University of California (buildings and grounds and student organizations), (7) business groups, (8) lay organizations (service clubs, women's clubs, etc.), (9) city recreation department, (10) exhibit and window-display groups, (11) press, (12) radio and movies. In addition, certain individuals were given special responsibility for (1) printed matter and visual materials, (2) exhibits and window displays, and (3) meetings.

The county medical society and the local dental association joined the project at the beginning. A demonstration of killing poison oak with 2,4-D was carried out on the university campus, the success of which was recorded in still and in moving pictures. The student-body put on an educational program of its own, as did the public schools. Twenty-five thousand "stuffers" were sent to citizens in monthly bills from the city and from public utilities. The press, the local radio station, the Boy Scouts, the service clubs, the women's clubs, and commercial interests all participated. As a result, an extensive spraying program got under way in local and regional parks, on university grounds, along the roadsides, and on the private property of many scores of individual citizens.

The City of Berkeley, through the leadership of the Park Department, has continued poison-oak eradication with splendid results. Medical cost for Rhus poisoning on the campus has been cut in half. The use of 2,4-D against poison ivy and poison oak has become fairly widespread, especially with groups having summer camp programs such as Boy Scouts, Girl Scouts and YMCA. The expansion of the California State Health Department program was accelerated by the accidental poisoning of the state health officer at the time the project was being considered.

# 32

## MANY VISITS TO LATIN AMERICA

In starting duties as Chief Health Education Officer for the Institute of Inter-American Affairs in February, 1944, the first three weeks were devoted to the intensive study of Spanish in the Washington office, before beginning visits to the twenty-one countries with which we had cooperative health programs. Argentina was the only Latin American country with which we did not have a cooperative program. You would not be interested in technical public health activities, but you may be interested in incidental happenings.

I remember especially my first trip in which I stopped overnight at Port au Spain and flew on the next day to Belem. The chief of party there said that they had a chain of hookworm clinics up the river and that he could put at my disposal a small boat with a crew of five Brazilian sailors if I would like to visit these clinics. Dr. Charles Wagley, now Professor of Anthropology at Columbia University, went with me on this most interesting and exciting trip.

The first day we were surprisingly out of sight of land because the mouth of the Amazon really is an arm of the sea. In the late afternoon our boat put in at the location of the first clinic. We ate and slept on the boat where we had an excellent cook, but in the evening we talked with the medical director of the clinic. The conversation between Charles and the doctor was in Portuguese, so I missed it. But at one point I said to Charles, "The only word I have understood is the word for bull. What is that all about?"

"This is interesting," said Charles. "There is only one draft animal within miles of here, and the question is, should the clinic hire him or hire three men to move bricks from the wharf up to the site of the new building? The cost is about the same."

The next morning the clinic was in session and I asked the privilege of talking with people in the waiting room. Charles volunteered to translate my conversation with a man waiting for treatment. The man remarked, "My little girl has this disease, and we have to save up some money before she can be treated."

"Please explain to him," I said to Charles, "that he does not understand. The doctor is free and the medicine is free."

"It is the North American who does not understand," the man replied. "For generations we on the river have known that one must eat weak food before taking that kind of medicine (laxative or purgative). If my daughter eats fried chicken *(pollo frito)*, she will die. I must buy her a baby chick to eat."

An interesting illustration of the fact that health education is a needed accompaniment of medical programs!

And there was the incident of the room in Sao Paulo. We had an engineer over there, and the chief of party wired him to please make a reservation for me. His conversation with the hotel clerk was as follows:

"I would like a room for Dr. Turner for Thursday night," said the engineer.

"Sorry, we are full up."

"Oh, but this man is down here from the United States."

"I don't care where he is from, we have no room."

"You don't understand. He is Dr. Turner, he's Lana Turner's father."

"Oh, we have a room."

And there was the trip from Santiago to Valparaiso with my former student Rigoberto Rios Castro. Halfway there on a lonely mountain road our automobile coughed and stopped. The chauffeur looked over the engine and crawled under the car, where he went to sleep. After a bit we discovered that he was sleeping and woke him to ask what was the trouble. He said the glass cup to hold gasoline on the way to the cylinders was cracked and we would have to wait till someone came by to help us. We were saved by finding some adhesive tape in my kit and using it to mend the cup.

Upon arrival at Valparaiso, Dr. Rios had a cold and I sent him to bed. The next morning I came down to the desk to send up some breakfast to him, and had one of the most common experiences of travelers in foreign countries. I was just getting thoroughly stuck in my poor Spanish when the girl behind the desk said, "I'm sorry, could you speak a bit of English?"

There were many experiences of special interest, like the flight over the Andes from Argentina to Chile, the visit to the Central American Health Education Association, a visit to a village high in the mountains in Peru on market day, visits in Mexico City with the Spanish publisher of my book, *Personal and Community Health,* and with many distinguished acquaintances in public health.

My last visit to Latin America was following the distribution of the Spanish preliminary draft of *Planning for Health Education in Schools.* The Spanish translation had been made by a capable translator at Unesco who was not, however, an expert in public health or in health education. Unesco authorities were quite correct in their belief that a visit by the author to the countries engaged in the study would be necessary to make any needed corrections in the manuscript. For example, in Chile I sat down with the health educator and three other members of the staff.

"We find several statements in your manuscript with which we do not agree," said he. "Do you want us to point them out to you?"

"That's exactly why I am here," I said.

"For example, look at paragraph 1, on page 17," he said.

I read it to him from the English copy.

He said, "Oh, we agree with that, but that is not what the Spanish edition says."

Our struggle with this problem has made me ready to give

friendly consideration to possible errors when reading translated articles of technical papers.

My visit to Mexico was in connection with the "Planning" book and was especially pleasant. It included a visit to many leaders of Mexican activities. One of these was Jaime Torres Bodet, then Minister of Education but formerly Director General of Unesco.

# 33

## "PLANNING FOR HEALTH EDUCATION IN SCHOOLS"

My activities in planning health education programs for public schools extended over about forty years. The first of these activities was as consultant to the Cleveland, Ohio public schools in 1926-1927. An arrangement was made for me to serve as consultant to the school system, going to Cleveland from M.I.T. for brief visits during the first semester, and remaining in Cleveland full time for the second half of the year.

This curriculum planning came about primarily because several agencies in the community had made their way into the schools for the teaching of different topics, including tuberculosis, nutrition and child care. Superintendent Jones found these interruptions disturbing, and said to the public health people, "If you will find someone who can advise us in developing a complete program, we will do the health teaching ourselves, including whatever is desirable." Their reply was that Malden, Mass. had developed a good and broad program and perhaps the man responsible for that could be brought to Cleveland as a consultant.

Cleveland had an excellent school system. We established a central committee under the chairmanship of the Assistant Superintendent of Schools. It included the chief school physician, the director of school nursing, the director of school dental service, the director of physical education, a teacher of biology, a nutritionist, and the psychologist in charge of curriculum development.

The committee procedure was to prepare a framework

for the health education program and a statement of objectives in terms of desirable knowledge, habits and attitudes. The methods and procedures in the different grades we thought could best be determined by teachers in those grades who would look at the total program and decide what could be done at the respective levels at which they were teaching. The superintendent selected a subcommittee of three teachers from each grade and arranged for each group to be released from their teaching program for two weeks in order to work on the health-education program. We began with the kindergarten teachers, placing the objectives proposed by the central committee before them, and asking them what could be done in kindergarten and by what methods. Their report was given to the subcommittee of first-grade teachers, along with the plans from the central committee, and that group was asked what could be done in grade one.

Following this basic procedure, subcommittees of teachers from each of the six grades in the elementary schools presented their suggestions on gradation, methods and procedures. The elementary-school outline was placed before a committee of junior high-school teachers, and they prepared recommendations for the teaching of health in the junior high school. These subcommittee reports were returned to the central committee for examination, clarification and approval.

By the end of May we had teaching outlines for each grade, K to 6 and for the junior high school. The program for each grade was printed separately and the Cleveland outlines were, I believe, the first teacher guides for health prepared and presented in this way. The outline was presented to our school principals and printed in quantity. Quantity printing of these outlines was important because enough copies were sold to more than pay for the cost of their preparation.

The next adventure in school health-education program planning was some time later, when I was asked to come to Illinois to help plan a state program of school health education being undertaken by the Joint Committe on School

Health representing the Department of Health, the Department of Public Instruction, and the Department of Registration and Education. A committee was organized in October, 1943, and I met with this broad statewide committee several times during the school year. In the summer of 1944 the State published *A Basic Plan for Health Education and the School Health Program.* About ninety persons representing twenty-nine agencies were involved in this planning activity.

While the Illinois committee was working, we were visited by Miss May Hare, the Health Education Coordinator of the Kansas State Board of Health. She asked whether I could serve her state, and upon returning home she took the initial steps for the appointment of a State Policy-Making Committee on Health Education. The breadth of approach of the Kansas committe was similar to that of the Illinois program. In 1945 the committee published *Health Education in Elementary and Secondary Schools* and *Health Education in Colleges.*

Meeting, thinking and planning with these state-wide committees and with their various subcommittees was stimulating and interesting. I remember a particular incident at a meeting of a Kansas subcommittee. A question had come up to which no one had an answer. There was a minute of embarrassing silence which was ended by a county superintendent saying, "Well, thank God for the problems. That's why we're here." Many times since then, when facing a trying situation, I have reminded myself that if there were no difficult questions there would be no need for professionally skilled persons.

There have been shorter periods of consulting service to public schools in Boston, Brockton and other cities, but the most important of such program-planning activities has been a United Nations consultancy with Unesco and WHO to set up a methodology helpful to countries, regions and cities in planning for health education in schools. This was a joint activity in which I was seconded to Unesco by WHO.

During the first few months of 1962 I took to Paris from

WHO all of their books and materials dealing with school health education. These publications I reviewed, along with those in the library of Unesco. From the available literature and from previous experience, a preliminary draft was made for submission to the member states of both WHO and Unesco, seeking their assistance in the production of a publication on how to plan school health education.

In scope this program related to healthful school living, school health services, health instruction, and school, home and community cooperation. Ninety-four countries participated in the project.

When the English copy of the preliminary draft was finished, it was mimeographed and sent to ministries of health and ministries of education in English-speaking member states, with an introductory letter from the Director General of Unesco and the Director General of WHO. I went through the Middle East and Far East to discuss the material with education and health authorities in Iran, India, Thailand, the Philippines, Taiwan and Japan. Subsequently the material was translated into French and Spanish, mimeographed, and sent to the countries speaking those languages. After the Spanish copies were sent out, I visited the Latin American countries. From these visits, from correspondence and from materials accumulated from the ninety-four countries between 1962 and the fall of 1964, a revision was made which was published by Unesco in English, French and Spanish under the title *Planning for Health Education in Schools*. It has since been published by individual countries or by national agencies in Japanese, Arabic, Italian, Chinese, Thai and Nepalese.

## CURRICULUM VITAE

### C. E. TURNER

A.B. (Bates), A.M. (Harvard), M.P.H. (Harvard), Ed.M. (B.U.), Sc.D. (Hon.) (Bates), Dr.P.H. (M.I.T.)

(For biographical statements see "Who's Who in America," "World Biography," "American Men of Science," "Leaders in American Science," "Who's Important in Medicine," "American Men of Medicine," "Who's Who in American Education," "Who's Who Among American Authors," "Who's Who in the East," "Who's Who in New England.")

### I. TEACHING

1. Types of teaching experience include teaching in
   An ungraded school (Harmony, Maine);
   A grammar school (St. Albans, Maine);
   A high school (Wellington, Maine);
   College (Bates College, Tufts College, Jackson College);
   Technical school (Massachusetts Institute of Technology, 1914-44);
   Dental school (Tufts Dental School, 1917-29);
   Medical school (Tufts Medical School, 1917-29);
   Schools of Public Health [Harvard-Technology School of Public Health (1914-22), the School of Public Health at the University of California (1945-46)].
2. Established first program leading to the M.P.H. degree with specialization in Health Education ever offered in a School of Public Health and taught first course in Health Education offered in such a school. (See catalogue

of the Harvard-M.I.T. School of Public Health, 1921-22.)

3. First Professor of Health Education at the School of Public Health at the University of California.
4. Lecturer, University of Hawaii, Calcutta University, University of the Philippines, China Central University.

## II. RESEARCH

1. Director, Malden Study in Health Education and Growth, 1921-31, involving (1) studies in the effect of health education upon knowledge, habits and attitudes, (2) the development of the first series of grade school text-books on the basis of a separate book for each grade prepared by three successive years of experimentation with each manuscript before publication, (3) studies in the significance and limitations of "underweight" in children, (4) studies of the extent and significance of intermittency in growth, (5) studies on seasonal fluctuation of growth, (6) rate of growth as a health index.
2. Studies in the biological and chemical changes involved in the self purification process of a polluted stream, 1914-15.
3. Consultant in the Test Room Studies of Employee Effectiveness at the Hawthorne Plant of the Western Electric Company, 1928-32, at the time when Elton Mayo was consultant to the same company in connection with an employee interviewing program. It has been characterized by Hare, Borgatta & Bales in their book on "Small Groups" by the following statement: "Although systematic observations of individual and group behavior in the factory had been made in the early part of the century by F. K. Taylor and other proponents of scientific management, the Western Electric researches, described here in an early article by Turner, are generally regarded as the classic studies in the industrial area of small group research." See Publication 11.

4. Studies in Community Organization for Health Education (with P. L. Riley), 1940-41.
5. A study for UNESCO and WHO with 94 countries on Planning for Health Education in Schools, 1962-65. See Publication 18.

## III. CONSULTANTSHIPS

1. Member of Advisory Education Group of the Metropolitan Life Insurance Company, 1924-1944.
2. Consultant in the development of school health education curricula: Cleveland, Ohio (1926-27), Illinois State Dept. of Health (1943-50), Kansas State Board of Health (1944-50), Boston Health Dept. (1941-46), City of Brockton (1938-39), Boston Parochial Schools (1943).
3. Consultant to Eastman Teaching Films of Eastman Kodak Company (1928-33) in the development of films for the teaching of health in public schools.
4. Consultant to the National Ministry of Health and Education, Nanking, China (1936).
5. Public Health Expert with Overseas Consultants, Incorporated, to the government of Iran in 1948-49 in laying the Seven Year Plan for that country.
6. Consultant to World Health Organization in 1949 in the establishment of the Section on Health Education of the Public, and subsequently on special projects.
7. Consultant to WHO and UNESCO (1951) concerning health education in Egypt and Iraq.
8. Chief Advisor, International Union for Health Education, 1956-68.
9. Technical Advisor in Health Education, League of Red Cross Societies, 1958-62.
10. Consultant to Expert Committee of WHO and UNESCO on the Teacher Preparation for Health Education, 1960-61.

## IV. ADMINISTRATION

1. Acting Head, Department of Biology, Bates College (1913-14).
2. Sanitary Engineer, 1st Lieutenant Grade, U.S. Public Health Service (1917-19).
3. Member Administrative Board, Harvard-M.I.T. School of Public Health (1921-22).
4. Major, Sanitary Corps Reserve, U.S. Army (1924-34).
5. Professor of Public Health and Head of the Department, Massachusetts Institute of Technology (1943-44).
6. Chief Health Education Officer, Institute of Inter-American Affairs (1944-45).
7. Assistant to the President, National Foundation for Infantile Paralysis (1946-58).
8. Chief, Health Education, World Health Organization (1962-64).

## V. SOME FORMER COLLEAGUES IN TEACHING AND PROFESSIONAL ACTIVITIES

W. T. Sedgwick, Milton Rosenau, G. C. Whipple, Selskar Gunn, C. E.-A. Winslow, E. O. Jordan, William Welch, Sally Lucas Jean, Mahidol, Prince of Songkla and Madam Mahidol, father and mother of the King of Siam.

## VI. HONORS AND AWARDS

1. Secretary (1919-23) and later Chairman (1924-32) APHA Sub-Committee on Training and Personnel. A Sub-Committee of the Committee on Research and Standards.
2. Trustee, Bates College (1922-1973).
3. Honorary President, New England Health Education Association (1924- ).
4. Chairman, Health Section, World Federation of Education Associations (1927-40).
5. Sc.D. (Honorary) Bates College (1927).

6. Member Governing Council, American Public Health Association (1928-30, 1942).
7. Member of the Executive Board, American Public Health Association (1928-29, 1933-35).
8. Member (1933-40), Chairman (1941-53) APHA Committee on Educational Qualifications of Community Health Educators.
9. Chairman, National Conference for Cooperation in Health Education (1938-42).
10. President, American School Health Association (1942-43).
11. Howe Award in School Health of the American School Health Association (1949).
12. First President, Society of Public Health Educators (1950-51).
13. First President (1951-56), Chief Advisor (1956-68), Honorary President (1968- ), of the International Union for Health Education.
14. Medal of the City of Paris (1953).
15. Prentiss Award (1953).
16. Recipient gold medal of the National Academy of Medicine, France (1958).
17. Great Cross of the Order of Merit, German Federal Republic (1959).
18. Associate Fellow, American Medical Association.
19. Fellow: American Academy of Arts and Sciences; American Academy of Physical Education; American Public Health Association; American School Health Association; American Association for Health, Physical Education & Recreation.
20. Honorary Fraternities: Phi Beta Kappa, Sigma Xi, Delta Sigma Rho, Delta Omega, Phi Delta Kappa.
21. Honorary Member Philippine Public Health Association.
22. Honorary Fellow, Society of Public Health Educators.
23. Ira V. Hiscock Award of the New England Public Health Association (1973).

24. First recipient of the Parisot Medal of the International Union for Health Education (1973).

## VII. PUBLICATIONS

1. *Studies on Digestion of a Sewage Filter Effluent in a Small and Otherwise Unpolluted Stream* (with Robert Spurr Weston) 114 pp., 1915.
2. *Hygiene, Dental and General,* 400 pp., 1920.
3. Health Education, A Course of Study, grades K through 9 (as consultant, for Cleveland Public Schools).
4. *Malden Health Series,* 8 books, Grades 2-9, 1924-37.
5. *Personal and Community Health.* First edition, 426 pp., 1925. Fourteenth edition, 1971. (Translated into Spanish.)
6. *Louis Pasteur* (with Grace T. Hallock) 238 pp., 1928.
7. *Edward Jenner* (with Grace T. Hallock) 204 pp., 1928.
8. *Edward Livingston Trudeau* (with Grace T. Hallock) 166 pp., 1929.
9. *School Health Appraisal Form,* 73 pp., 1920.
10. *Principles of Health Education,* 1932. (Translated into Chinese and Japanese.)
11. *Test Room Studies in Employee Effectiveness,* AJPH, 8 pp., June 1933.
12. *Personal Hygiene,* 335 pp., 1937.
13. *Community Organization for Health Education* (with a committee) 120 pp., 1941.
14. *Effective Living* (with Elizabeth McHose) 432 pp., 1941, 3 editions.
15. *Health, Safety, Growth Series,* 6 books, Grades 4-9, 1941.
16. *School Health and Health Education,* 1947. (Translated into Japanese), Ed. 6, 1970.
17. *Check* (Community Health Educators Compendium of Knowledge), 259 pp., 1951. (Translated into French by Annette Le Meitour Kaplun), 1973.
18. *Planning for Health Education in Schools,* 1966, 157 pp., published jointly by UNESCO and WHO in Eng-

lish, French, and Spanish. Published separately in Japanese, Arabic, Chinese, Siamese, Nepalese and Italian.

19. *I Remember,* 1973.
20. Over 100 articles in professional periodicals.

## VIII. COUNTRIES VISITED

Canada, Mexico, Guatemala, Honduras, Nicaragua, Costa Rica, Panama, Colombia, Equador, Peru, Chile, Bolivia, Argentina, Uruguay, Paraguay, Brazil, Guiana, Venezuela, Cuba, Dominican Republic, Haiti, Jamaica, Bahama, England, Scotland, Ireland, Portugal, Spain, France, Germany, Belgium, The Netherlands, Iceland, Greenland, Denmark, Norway, Sweden, Finland, U.S.S.R., Poland, Czechoslovakia, Hungary, Switzerland, Yugoslavia, Italy, Austria, Greece, Turkey, Syria, Iraq, Iran, Jordan, Israel, Egypt, Aden, India, Burma, Thailand, Malaya, French Indo China, Java, Bali, Celebes, Borneo, The Philippines, China, Manchuria, Japan, Korea, Taiwan, Nigeria, Congo, Cameroons, Lebanon, Monaco, Luxembourg, and E. Germany.